T0220686

THE MINDFUL BRAIN

THE MINDFUL BRAIN

Cortical Organization and the
Group-Selective Theory of
Higher Brain Function

Gerald M. Edelman

Vernon B. Mountcastle

Introduction
by
Francis O. Schmitt

The MIT Press
Cambridge, Massachusetts, and London, England

These essays derive from presentations at the Fourth Intensive Study Program of the Neurosciences Research Program, held on 20 June through 1 July 1977 in Boulder, Colorado. They will also be included in the resulting volume *The Neurosciences: Fourth Study Program.*

Sponsored by the Massachusetts Institute of Technology, the Neurosciences Research Program is supported in part by U.S. Public Health Service, National Institutes of Health Contract No. NO1-NS-6-2343, National Institute of Mental Health Grant No. NIH-5-RO1-MH23132-05, National Science Foundation Grant No. 76-08344-BNS, The Arthur Vining Davis Foundation, William T. Grant Foundation, van Ameringen Foundation, Inc., Vingo Trust, and the Neurosciences Research Foundation, Inc.

Grateful acknowledgement for direct support of the Intensive Study Program is made to the following: National Institutes of Health Contract No. 278-77-0009 (ER), National Science Foundation, International Business Machine Corp., Vollmer Foundation, Inc., Surdna Foundation, Inc., The Teagle Foundation, Inc., The National Foundation, and the Camille and Henry Dreyfus Foundation, Inc.

First MIT Press paperback edition, 1982

Copyright © 1978 by The Massachusetts Institute of Technology

This book was set in IBM Composer Press Roman by Eastern Composition, Inc.

Library of Congress Cataloging in Publication Data

Edelman, Gerald M.
  The mindful brain.

  Based on papers presented at the fourth intensive study program of the Neurosciences Research Program, held in June 1977.
  Bibliography: p.
  1. Higher nervous activity. 2. Neural circuitry. 3. Cerebral cortex. 4. Brain. I. Mountcastle, Vernon B., joint author. II. Neurosciences Research Program. III. Title. [DNLM: 1. Brain—Physiology. 2. Cerebral cortex—Physiology. WL300.3 E21m]
QP395.E36   153   78-4604

ISBN 978-0-262-05020-3 (hc : alk. paper), 978-0-262-55007-9 (pb)

CONTENTS

CONTENTS

INTRODUCTION

Francis O. Schmitt

Neuroscience, the multidisciplinary study of the central nervous system, has expanded greatly during the last two decades both in numbers of investigators and in subjects being investigated at all levels of complexity, from that of molecules, brain cells, and brain systems to that of behavior. New discoveries and conceptual advances enliven the meetings of national and international societies of neuroscience. Highly sophisticated concepts of the function of various partial systems of the brain have been developed on the basis of ingenious experimental designs in anatomy, physiology, and other aspects of neuroscience. These advances are valuable and meaningful not only in their own right but as a basic foundation for a scientifically significant attempt to understand the most complex known mechanism, the human brain, and to achieve the highest ultimate aim, a comprehension of human selfhood and psyche.

Many theories of higher brain function (learning, memory, perception, self-awareness, consciousness) have been proposed; but in general these lack cogency with respect to established anatomical and physiological facts and are without biophysical and biochemical plausibility.

These theories usually rely heavily upon processes subserved by spike action potential waves traveling in hard-wired circuits of Golgi Type I neurons. Such circuits consist of neurons that are large enough to permit easy impalement by microelectrodes and that possess long axons forming tracts connecting processing centers in general regions of the brain that have been characterized as sensory, motor, associational, frontal, temporal, parietal, and occipital.

Theories based on partial systems are subject, however, to the component-systems dilemma that bedevils all attempts at biological generalization. Such theories fail to articulate and effectively deal with the essence of the problem, which is the distributive aspect that emerges from the complex interaction of functional units such as neurons or neuronal circuits in the brain. Until now no detailed, self-consistent theory has been proposed that specifies and functionally characterizes the operational repertoires at the level of molecules, individual neurons, or groups (circuits) of neurons and that explicitly defines the postulated information-processing mechanism.

To add another increment to the basic substructure of neuroscience on which a theory of higher brain function might be built, the Neurosciences Research Program (NRP) held a two-week Intensive Study Program (ISP) in June of 1977, the fourth in a series that began in 1966. Emphasis was placed on "local circuits," composed primarily, but not exclusively, of small Golgi II neurons. These small cells are very numerous in the brain and have short, although sometimes bushy, axons that do not extend into major tracts of white matter beyond the local area. At this ISP there was much discussion of neuronal local circuits in the sense defined by Rakic (1975). These are characterized by extensive dendrodendritic synaptic interaction and by graded electrotonic processing such as occurs in the retina, an externalized bit of central nervous system that serves as an example par excellence of neuronal local circuits.

As was pointed out by Theodore Bullock and Floyd Bloom in their 1977 ISP lectures, the purpose of the ISP was more general than might be inferred from the term "local circuits," narrowly defined. It was concerned with integrative processes, whether intracellular (as by intramembranous molecular differentiations) or in localized groupings of neurons.

In his keynote, Professor Vernon Mountcastle discussed the columnar organizations of the cerebral cortex. He postulated that the manner in which local cortical columns, as processing and distributing units, operate upon their inputs to produce their outputs is qualitatively similar in all neocortical areas and is basic to the carrying out of high-order functions by the brain. The essence of his lecture was that, although phylogenetically older parts of the brain may play a significant role, the key to any fruitful theories of higher brain function must be the unique structure and properties of the cerebral cortex.

At this point in the scenario of the ISP, it was thought that a theoretical approach to the problem of higher brain function might be usefully introduced. Professor Gerald Edelman had on many occasions lectured to his fellow NRP Associates on concepts significant for neurobiological theory arising from current developments in immunobiological and immunochemical research, a theme that had been touched on briefly at the 1966 ISP. But such notions of the applicability of selectionist—as contrasted with instructionist—theories to neurobiology were articulated only in a very general manner; they were not at that time elaborated into a detailed, self-consistent theory capable of confirmation or falsification by known fact or crucial experiment.

In more recent years, as Edelman has more actively pursued problems basic to neurobiology, there took shape in his mind in increasingly precise form an ingenious theory of higher brain function. This began to crystallize in a clearly articulated form just as final planning was proceeding for the 1977 ISP. He had agreed to organize and chair a one-day section on membrane dynamics and cellular interaction and to give a lead paper of his own on cell surface modulation and transmembrane control.

At a meeting on January 7, 1977, with ISP section chairmen, a meaningful way was sought, in programming the last ISP afternoon, to project the lessons learned about the properties and role in brain function of local neuronal circuits and local integrative processes. The most exciting and rather daring plan, and the one finally adopted, was to devote that afternoon to a full presentation by Edelman of his theory. After reading a preliminary version of Edelman's manuscript and discussing it with him in detail, Mountcastle agreed to chair the last afternoon program and to introduce Edelman's lecture with relevant remarks taken from his own keynote lecture.

It is perhaps desirable at this point to demonstrate the close interrelationship of the two viewpoints, the convergence of theory with experimentally established facts, by conveying very briefly the essence of both Mountcastle's and Edelman's contributions. In this monograph, Edelman's paper is given essentially as it was presented on July 1, 1977, copies having been distributed to all participants on the previous day. Mountcastle's paper is based on his keynote lecture but amplified to bring out the generalizable concepts that can be deduced from the major facts.

Mountcastle proposes that higher functions depend on the ensemble actions of very large populations of neurons in the forebrain, organized into complex interaction systems. To focus on those properties of the cerebral cortex that are of fundamental importance for concepts of higher brain function, Mountcastle points to the fantastically large population of neurons in the neocortex of the forebrain, which are organized in multiply replicated local neuronal circuits constituting *columns*, which, in turn, are composed of closely linked subsets or *minicolumns*. Columns, which may comprise hundreds to thousands of neurons, are composed of both Golgi I neurons in conventional synaptic patterns and the local circuit, Golgi II neurons described by Rakic (1975), the possible significance of which was the subject of a paper by Schmitt, Dev, and Smith (1976) and of a large share of the 1977 ISP.

In various parts of the cortex, the shape of the columns may vary due to the number and mode of packing of the constituent minicolumns. It is the columns that are pictured as the fundamental local units. The neocortex is pictured as being everywhere much more uniform than has hitherto been supposed; the avalanche of phylogenetic enlargement in primates occurred by replication of basically similar columns rather than by the development of new neuronal types or different modes of intrinsic organization. Intracolumnar and intercolumnar connections are precisely arrayed, but they constitute *distributed systems* serving *distributive functions*. The cortex is composed of a repetitive, pervasive, internal structure that is everywhere the same.

The neocortex, which receives afferent input upon the intracortical columns, has outputs to almost every major entity of the CNS, many of them forming massive reentrant systems with many points of entry and exit.

The uninitiated reader may well be surprised by two aspects of Mountcastle's description: first, the counts of Powell and his colleagues (Rockel, Hiorns, and Powell, 1974) show the apparent precision with which the dimensions and the number of the neurons contained within a narrow cortical cylinder can be specified (about 110 neurons in all mammals studied, except for 260 in the striate cortex of primates); and, second, the 600 million minicolumns of the human cortex are composed of about 50 billion nerve cells. It has been only about a decade since most textbooks put the total population of the entire brain at 10 billion neurons.

The enormity of this number is not merely a matter of passing note in Mountcastle's paper; and it is vital for the argument of Edelman, who points to the fact that the number of neuronal groups is of the same order of magnitude as the variants possible in the gamma globulin macromolecule that subserve immune phenomena. This is in agreement with his view that the substrates of higher brain function, like immunological processes, interact selectionistically.

Besides the strikingly large numbers of neurons involved and the repetitive nature of their organization into local groups (columns and their constituent minicolumns), Mountcastle strongly emphasizes a second fact that is also fundamental to Edelman's concept—that each of the basic, unitary subsets of which the neocortex is composed is linked by patterns of connections to similar columnar subsets in other brain regions to form distributed systems that are reentrant, structurally and functionally. This fits well with Edelman's hypothesis that the phasic cycling of internally generated activity by this organization may facilitate continual updating of the perceptual image of the self.

The most striking aspect of Edelman's theory is that it is thoroughly and rigidly selectionistic; incoming sensory signals play no role in forming the basic anatomical connections that make up the primary repertoire. The selectional operational units are groups, each composed of hundreds or thousands of neurons which constitute the local units ("primary repertoire") and which are present in vast numbers in the cortex. Mountcastle's columnar units and minicolumn subsets fit this description perfectly. The local neuronal groups form the primary repertoire analogous, although not homologous, to the nucleotide codons of the genetic code. The intrinsic and extrinsic neuronal circuitry within and between the unitary clusters is specified genetically and ontogenetically. The repertoire of neuronal groups, columns, or modules permits matching of repertoire groups to sensory signals in a degenerate manner, that is, with more than one way by which the repertoire can recognize given input signals. The concept of degeneracy differs from redundancy, which characterizes *identical* structures.

"Recognition" of unitary groups is by electrical, ultrastructural, and connectionistic action and is precise. Multiple signaling to primary repertoire groups leads to associative recognition and the formation of a *secondary repertoire* of neuronal groups having a higher likelihood of response than the cell groups of the primary repertoire.

As a result of experience and the formation of secondary repertoires, structures are formed that discriminate between self inputs and external inputs.

Consciousness, it is hypothesized, may result from reentrant signaling that involves associations between current sensory input and stored patterns of neuronal groups. Details are specified about the stages in which reentrant signals are processed in relation to responses in primary and secondary repertoires.

It is important to emphasize that the concept of reentry is a critical one. Because of the degenerate nature of the proposed selection process, the absence of reentry would lead to a failure of continuity in the system as well as a failure to form coordinated abstract representations of external signals. In other words, reentry guarantees continuity in a distributed selectional system. Consciousness may be a kind of associative recollective updating by reentrant inputs that continually confirms or alters the theory of the self by parallel sensory or motor inputs and outputs.

The degree to which the papers of Mountcastle and Edelman complement each other, although evident when the papers were presented, is much more strikingly obvious in the full manuscripts. They will, of course, be included in the large volume, *The Neurosciences: Fourth Study Program*, that will harvest the proceedings of the 1977 ISP. However, to accentuate the communality and the complementarity of the message that is conveyed by the pair and to make the work more easily accessible to a large and diverse readership, it was thought appropriate to publish them together in this volume.

References

Rakic, P., 1975. *Local Circuit Neurons (Neurosci. Res. Program Bull.* 13, no. 2). Cambridge, Mass.: The MIT Press.

Rockel, A.J., R.W. Hiorns, and T.P.S. Powell, 1974. Numbers of neurons through full depth of neocortex. *Proc. Anat. Soc. Gr. Br. Ire.* 118:371.

Schmitt, F.O., P. Dev, and B.H. Smith, 1976. Electronic processing of information by brain cells. *Science* 193:114–120.

Schmitt, F.O., and F.G. Worden, eds., 1978. *The Neurosciences. Fourth Study Program.* Cambridge, Mass.: The MIT Press.

AN ORGANIZING PRINCIPLE FOR CEREBRAL FUNCTION: THE UNIT MODULE AND THE DISTRIBUTED SYSTEM

Vernon B. Mountcastle

Introduction

There can be little doubt of the dominating influence of the Darwinian revolution of the mid-nineteenth century upon concepts of the structure and function of the nervous system. The ideas of Spencer and Jackson and Sherrington and the many who followed them were rooted in the evolutionary theory that the brain develops in phylogeny by the successive addition of more cephalad parts. On this theory each new addition or enlargement was accompanied by the elaboration of more complex behavior and, at the same time, imposed a regulation upon more caudal and primitive parts and the presumably more primitive behavior they control. Dissolution of this hierarchy is thought to be revealed by disease or lesions of the brain in humans and by lesions or truncation of the neuraxis in experimental animals. The importance of these ideas can scarcely be exaggerated; for nearly a century they dominated the theory and practice of brain research, and experiments based on them yielded much of our present knowledge of the nervous system. They retained vigor and influence into the 1950s and still form a base for further advance in many fields of neuroscience.

Developments of recent decades require new formulations that include but transcend the hierarchical principle of brain organization. Prominent among them is the concept that the brain is a complex of widely and reciprocally interconnected systems and that the dynamic interplay of neural activity within and between these systems is the very essence of brain function. The large entities of advanced brains and their gross and microscopic inter- and intra-system connections have developed in phylogeny in accord, it is thought, with evolutionary principles. They are determined genetically, but at the level of ultrastructure and of molecular events they are to some extent modifiable by postnatal experience. These entities are so widely, reciprocally, divergently and convergently (but specifically) interconnected, and the ongoing activity within the systems they compose is so pervasive and continuous, that—particularly as regards the cerebral hemispheres—the hierarchical principle expressed by such antonyms as higher–lower or newer–older loses some of its heuristic value.

7

I present below a set of ideas that in sum compose an organizing principle or paradigm for cerebral function. It builds upon knowledge gained from experiments based upon evolutionary theory and its hierarchical principle, and it also includes the concept of the brain as a dynamic information-processing machine. More subtle and complex aspects of behavior are generally thought of as initiated and controlled by "higher" levels of the neuraxis: particularly perceiving, remembering, thinking, calculating, formulating plans for current and future action, and consciousness itself. I regard them as depending upon—that is, as the internally experienced and sometimes externally observable behavioral events produced by—the ensemble actions of large populations of neurons of the forebrain, organized into complex interacting systems. No external influences incompatible with the presently known laws of thermodynamics are imagined to exist. The principle is thus exactly consonant with that of Psychoneural Identity and exactly opposed to that of Cartesian Dualism, whether in its original or its more recent formulations.

The general idea is as follows. The large entities of the brain we know as areas (or nuclei) of the neocortex, the limbic lobe, basal ganglia, dorsal thalamus, and so forth, are themselves composed of replicated *local neural circuits*, modules which vary in cell number, intrinsic connections, and processing mode from one large entity to another but are basically similar within any given entity (Szentágothai and Arbib, 1974; Szentágothai, 1975). Each module is a local neural circuit that processes information from its input to its output and in that processing imposes transforms determined by the general properties of the entity and its extrinsic connections. Modules are grouped into entities such as nuclei or cortical areas by a common or dominating extrinsic connection, by the need to replicate a function over a topographic representation, or by some other factor. The set of modules composing an entity may itself be fractionated into subsets by different linkages to similarly segregated subsets in other large entities. Closely linked and multiply interconnected subsets of modules in different and often widely separated entities thus form precisely connected but distributed systems. The preservation of neighborhood relations between the interconnected subsets of topographically organized entities results in nested distributed systems. *Such a distributed system is conceived to serve a distributed function.* A single module of an entity may be a member of several (but not many) such systems. Only in the limiting case might all the modules of an entity have identical connections.

I wish to explore these ideas, particularly as regards the neocortex, and the general proposition that the processing function of neocortical modules is qualitatively similar in all neocortical regions. Put shortly, there is nothing intrinsically motor about the motor cortex, nor sensory about the sensory cortex. Thus the elucidation of the mode of operation of the local modular circuit anywhere in the neocortex will be of great generalizing significance. This idea is unrelated to the equipotentiality concept of Lashley (1949).

I shall start with a brief résumé of what is known of the phylogenetic and ontogenetic development of the neocortex and its cytoarchitecture, facts which I believe are consonant with the general hypothesis.

Phylogenetic Development of the Neocortex

The avalanching enlargement of the neocortex is a major aspect of mammalian evolution and, in its degree, distinguishes primates from other mammals and man from other primates. A major goal of comparative neurology is to reconstruct the evolutionary development of man's brain by measuring both the endocranial casts of fossils and the brains of living primates and their putative insectivore ancestors (Jerison, 1973). Brain measurements in living primates are valuable for such a reconstruction largely by retrospective inference, for a salient feature of primate evolution is its parallel and radiating nature (Washburn and Harding, 1970; Hodos, 1970). For example, the living primates readily available for neurological research in significant numbers, the new and the old world monkeys, diverged from the line leading to man (and from each other) more than 30 million years ago. However, detailed measurements of the total brain and of the relative sizes of different brain parts in insectivores, prosimians, and simians do provide an ordinal ranking of species in terms of brain development, and the degree of brain development provides the best available correlation with the evolutionary level of achievement. Moreover, the careful measurements of Stephan and his colleagues (Stephan, 1967, 1969, 1972; Stephan and Andy, 1964, 1969; Stephen, Bauchot, and Andy, 1970) in more than sixty species have revealed that, of all cerebral parts, it is the absolute and relative development of the neocortex that correlates best with evolutionary achievement.

The living basal insectivores are thought to have evolved very little from their ancestors, from which man's line also arose. Stephan has used this fact to establish an index of the evolutionary development of a brain structure as the ratio of its observed volume to that expected in a basal insectivore of the same body weight. The progression index for neocortex is 156 for man, 60 for chimpanzee, and 40 for Cercopithecidae. Some unusual ratios occasionally occur when such an allometric method is used; for example, the high rank of miopithecus is thought to be due to secondary body dwarfing, while the low rank of the gorilla may be due to body gigantism. These aberrations disappear when the volume of neocortex is related to the area of the foramen magnum (Radinsky, 1967) or to the volume of the medulla (Sacher, 1970). The degree of differential development of the neocortex in man is emphasized by the progression indices for different brain parts: neocortex, 156; striatum, 17; hippocampus, 4; cerebellum, 5; dorsal thalamus, 5; basal olfactory structures and olfactory bulb, 1 or less.

The progressive development of neocortex in primates is not uniform over its entire extent. For example, although the striate area is strongly progressive in prosimians, it is much less so in simians and especially in man, where it is reduced relative to overall neocortex. The striate area is not well defined in insectivores, and for this reason Stephan (1969) used the lepilemur as a base against which to measure the progression of this region, for this prosimian possesses the smallest clearly defined striate area. On this basis, the progression index for the striate area in man is less than one-fourth that of the neocortex as a whole. If the relative development of other sensory cortical areas is similar, one may infer that the progression index for the eulaminate homotypical cortex is even higher than the figure of 156 given for the total neocortex in man.

The enlargement of the neocortex in primates has been accomplished by a great expansion of its surface area, without striking changes in vertical organization. Indeed, Powell and his colleagues have shown that the number of neurons in a vertical line across the thickness of the cortex—that is, in a 30-μm-diameter cylinder—is remarkably constant at about 110 (Rockel, Hiorns, and Powell, 1974). The counts are virtually identical for the five areas studied in five species: the motor, somatic sensory, and frontal, parietal, and temporal homotypical cortices in the mouse, cat, rat, macaque monkey, and man. There is somewhat more than a doubling of the count in the striate cortex of most primates, for which no ready explanation is available.

Although with the one exception noted the number of cells in a small cylinder of neocortex is invariant, the packing density does differ.

The thickness of the cortex, the height of that small cylinder, varies by a factor of about three in different mammals, and there are some differences in thickness from one area to another in the same brain. It seems very likely that these differences are due to variations in the development of dendritic trees and synaptic neuropil (Bok, 1959). On the basis of electron-microscopic evidence, the ratio of the two main classes of neurons, the pyramidal and stellate cells, remains at about 2 to 1 in such diverse cytoarchitectural and functional areas as the motor, somatic sensory, and visual areas in the macaque (Sloper, 1973; Tömböl, 1974) and in the rat and cat (Gatter, Winfield, and Powell, 1977). A number of subtypes of these two major classes of cells have been described, but the appearance of new subtypes is not correlated with the evolutionary trend of neocortex, and it is unlikely that at any particular stage of mammalian evolution wholly new cell types have appeared that are unique to one brain as compared with other presumably more primitive or simpler ones.

Ontogenetic Development of the Neocortex

The ontogenetic development of the primate neocortex has been clarified by the work of a number of investigators using the radioactive labeling of dividing cells (for review, see Sidman, 1970) and, in the present context, particularly by the studies of Rakic in the monkey (Rakic, 1971, 1972, 1974, 1975, 1978; Sidman and Rakic, 1973). All of the cells destined for the neocortex of the macaque monkey arise from the ventricular and subventricular zones of the neural tube during the two-month period between the 45th and the 102nd day of the 165-day gestational period. Those cells destined for successively more superficial laminae arise in a regularly ordered temporal sequence: the neocortex is constructed from "inside to outside." Cells that arise early, mainly from the ventricular zone, may move over their short migratory trajectories of 200 to 300 μm by extension of a process and nuclear translocation. Cells arising later must migrate over distances of up to 10 mm; they are guided to their final positions by moving along the surfaces of radially oriented glial cells which extend across the entire wall of the neural tube. The result is that the cortical cells are arranged in radially oriented cords or columns extending across the cortex, and it has been suggested that the cells of such a column constitute a single clonal derivative (Meller and Tetzlaff, 1975). The special glial cells have

been studied in detail by Rakic (1971, 1972) and by Schmechel and
Rakic (1973). They can be identified in the monkey by the 70th day of
gestation, after neuronal migration begins. They begin to decrease in
number by the 120th day, two weeks after migration is complete, and
thereafter show transitional forms.

From the data provided by these studies of neocortical development and an examination of a series of fetal brains (Powell and
Mountcastle, 1977), it can be said that the cytoarchitectural differences
characteristic of the neocortex of the newborn and the adult primate
have not appeared at the time in fetal development when all the cortical
cells have reached their final positions. Clear cytoarchitectural features
can be recognized by E-108, a week after the generation of the last
cortical cells, at the time when the fibers from the lateral geniculate
nucleus are just reaching the cortex (Rakic, 1977). Area 17 has then become almost as distinct and sharply delimited as it is in the adult brain.
Its boundaries lie along the banks of a calcarine sulcus whose depth has
increased remarkably during the preceding 10 days. There is less
marked but suggestive architectonic differentiation in other parts of
the neocortex of the monkey at this stage on E-108. One example is
seen between areas 3 and 4 in the walls of an incipient central sulcus.
It thus appears that the intrinsic morphological differentiation of the
neocortex begins immediately after the stage at which the cortical cells
have reached their final position. Examination of fetal material has confirmed the finding of Rakic that at this stage of development the cells
of the cortex are clearly arranged in columns.

Are Cytoarchitectural Differences Causally Related to Differences in the Function of Different Cortical Areas?

Even brief inspection of serial sections reveals that there are differences in intrinsic structure between different regions of the cerebral
cortex, particularly in the neocortex. The development of the field of
cytoarchitectonics began with Meynert and is associated with the names
of Campbell, Broadmann, Elliott Smith, von Economo, and the Vogts.
Their efforts and the work of many who followed them resulted in detailed parcellations and hence maps of the cerebral cortex in a number
of mammals, including man, based upon variations in the numbers and
packing densities of cells of different types and sizes in homologous
layers of different cortical regions. In some cases other criteria were

used, such as the degree and temporal sequence of myelination of intrinsic or extrinsic nerve fibers. When pushed to the extreme by those sophisticated in its use, even minute parcellations of the cerebral cortex were thought to be valid. Some cytoarchitectonicists and neurologists of that era took the position that these morphologically identified regions were to be regarded as quasi-independent cerebral "organs," each functioning independently of its neighbors; this point of view has not been argued seriously for half a century. A period of sharp controversy followed the early years of cytoarchitectural study; the reaction against detailed parcellation was so great that some regarded all but the most obvious differences between cortical areas as subjective impressions (Lashley and Clark, 1946; Bonin and Bailey, 1947).

These old controversies now seem to be settled. There is general agreement that structural differences do exist between major regions of neocortex and that these differences can be defined objectively. They are a regular feature of the neocortex of any given species, and the areas so specified can be homologized over a series of mammals. Equally certain is the fact that cytoarchitecturally different cortical regions subserve different functions, where the term "function" takes its ordinary and usual sense (for example, the control of movement or the primary processing of a sensory input). That at least is the conclusion one must draw from nearly a century of study of the effects produced by electrical stimulation of the neocortex and of the behavioral changes that follow lesions confined to one or another of the major cytoarchitectural fields within it. This conclusion has been greatly strengthened by recent neuroanatomical studies, especially those in which new methods for defining connectivity have been used (important contributions have been made by Nauta, Powell, Jones, Kuypers, Akert, and others). One can now conclude that each neocortical area that has a distinctive cytoarchitecture and a distinctive "function" also possesses a unique set of extrinsic connections, that is, its own pattern of thalamic, corticocortical, interhemispheric, and long descending connections. Thus a major question concerning the neocortex is this: *To what degree are the three variables of cytoarchitecture, extrinsic connections, and "function" causally related?* It should be added that little is known of a possible fourth variable: differences in intrinsic microconnectivity in different cortical areas.

The discovery of the spontaneous electrical activity of the cerebral cortex led to the question of whether cortical areas defined cytoarchitecturally display differences in the pattern of electrical activity

recorded on the cortical surface or from an overlying spot on the scalp.
It was discovered that the electroencephalograms of very large regions
such as the frontal, parietal, and occipital lobes are indeed quite different, but no characteristic differences have been found between re-
cords from areas within those larger regions, which are clearly and
sometimes strikingly different in structural organization. Until now, at
least, study of the spontaneous slow-wave activity of the neocortex
has revealed little of its intrinsic functional organization.

A successful combination of descriptive cytoarchitecture and
experimental analysis was first made in a series of studies by Rose and
Woolsey. They found, for example, that the areas of the limbic cortex
of the cat and rabbit upon which the three anterior nuclei of the dorsal
thalamus project are clearly separated from one another by cytoarchitectural criteria and that each area thus defined receives the total projection of one nucleus and no other, with a narrow zone of transition
between areas (Rose and Woolsey, 1948a). A similar coincidence was
found between the orbitofrontal cortex of the cat defined by its intrinsic structure and the cortical projection zone of the mediodorsal
nucleus of the thalamus (Rose and Woolsey, 1948b). These same investigators added a third and independent method for defining the
extent of a cortical field in their study of the auditory cortex of the cat
(Rose, 1949; Rose and Woolsey, 1949). Here the three methods of
definition—cytoarchitecture, the cortical zone of projection of the
medial geniculate nucleus of the dorsal thalamus, and the area of cortex
activated by electrical stimulation of the spiral osseous lamina of the
cochlea—produced virtually coincident definitions of the auditory cortex. This led to the general conclusion that a cortical area may be defined both by its intrinsic structure and as the zone of projection of a
specific thalamic nucleus. This generality has since been confirmed in a
large number of studies in many species, including primates (Jones and
Burton, 1976; Jones and Wise, 1977). The results of more recent electrophysiological studies using single-unit analysis have strengthened this
idea considerably, for it has been shown that both the static and the
dynamic functional properties of cortical neurons can be correlated
with the cytoarchitectural area in which they are located. This has been
established in lightly anesthetized, unanesthetized but immobilized,
and waking, behaving monkeys, in the somatic sensory (Powell and
Mountcastle, 1959; Mountcastle and Powell, 1959a, b; Carli, LaMotte,
and Mountcastle, 1971a, b; Mountcastle et al., 1969), the visual (Hubel
and Wiesel, 1968, 1970, 1974a, b; Poggio et al., 1975; Poggio, Doty,

and Talbot, 1977; Poggio and Fischer, 1977), the motor (Evarts, 1964, 1974), and the association areas (Duffy and Birchfiel, 1972; Lynch et al., 1973a, b; Sakata et al., 1973; Hyvärinen and Poranen, 1974; Mountcastle et al., 1975; Lynch et al., 1977).

In summary, I conclude that cytoarchitectural differences between areas of neocortex reflect differences in their patterns of extrinsic connections. These patterns are in no way accidental. They are detailed and precise for each area; indeed, they define it. The traditional or usual "functions" of different areas also reflect these differences in extrinsic connections; they provide no evidence whatsoever for differences in *intrinsic* structure or function. This suggests that neocortex is everywhere functionally much more uniform than hitherto supposed and that its avalanching enlargement in mammals and particularly in primates has been accomplished by replication of a basic neural module, without the appearance of wholly new neuron types or of qualitatively different modes of intrinsic organization. Cytoarchitectural differences may therefore reflect the selection or grouping together of sets of modules in particular areas by certain sets of input-output connections. In the primary motor and sensory cortices this selection is made by a single strongly dominant connection, and cytoarchitectural identification of heterotypical areas is clear and striking. Areas of the homotypical eulaminate cortex (95% of man's neocortex) are defined by more evenly balanced sets of extrinsic connections, and here cytoarchitectural differences, while clear, are less striking. Thus a major problem for understanding the function of the neocortex and therefore of the cerebrum is to unravel the intrinsic structural and functional organization of the neocortical module.

That module is, I propose, what has come to be called the *cortical column*.

The Columnar Organization of the Cerebral Cortex

It was von Economo, I believe, who first used the world "column" to describe the vertical alignment of neurons in rows extending across all the cellular layers of the cortex. So far as I know, von Economo made no statement concerning the functional organization of the cortex, and it was Lorente de Nó who first suggested a vertical model of cortical operation, an idea to which he was led from his own Golgi studies of intracortical connectivity. The idea of the columnar organization of the cortex has developed as a functional concept on the basis of a discovery made in physiological experiments, namely that the basic unit of operation in the neocortex is a vertically arrayed group of cells heavily interconnected along that vertical axis, sparsely so horizontally. This unit is envisaged to function in the operations of processing and distribution. I emphasize again [for my earlier statements see Mountcastle (1957) and Powell and Mountcastle (1959)] that on this theory the cortex is, nevertheless, not regarded as a collection of isolated units cemented together in a mosaic, as some authors infer (Towe, 1975; Creutzfeldt, 1976). In the sections below I give some of the physiological evidence for this hypothesis and then call attention to some of the many important new discoveries concerning the intrinsic structure and connectivity of the neocortex that lend strong support to the columnar hypothesis. First, however, I list a number of relevant general principles that will be illustrated in what follows:

1. The cortical column is an input-output processing device. The number of other regions transmitting to and receiving from a traditionally defined cortical area may vary from about 10 to 30. The sample of that total entertained by any given subset of the modules of an area is much smaller and varies among subsets, with overlap.

2. The columnar arrangement allows the mapping of several variables simultaneously in a two-dimensional matrix.

3. Specific connections are maintained between ordered sets of columns in different cortical areas and between sets of cortical columns and modules of subcortical structures. Thus topological relations may be preserved during transit through and between such areas, with or without topographic (geographic) mapping.

4. The identification parameters for columns and ordered sets of columns may vary within a given cortical region, as defined traditionally, and may differ strikingly between cortical regions.

5. The columnar functional model allows for a partially shifted overlap across a topographical representation that is compatible with a dynamic isolation of the active elements of a column by a form of lateral, pericolumnar, inhibition.

6. Divergent intracolumnar pathways to different outputs allow selective processing ("feature extraction") of certain input signal parameters for particular output destinations.

Evidence from Study of the Somatic Sensory Cortex

Study of the first somatic sensory area of anesthetized cats produced evidence that the basic functional unit of the neocortex is a vertically oriented column (or cylinder, or slab) of cells which extends across all the cellular layers. Such a column is capable of input-output functions of considerable complexity, independently of horizontal spread of activity within the gray matter (Mountcastle, 1957). This hypothesis was confirmed and extended in studies of the homologous cortical area in anesthetized monkeys (Powell and Mountcastle, 1959). The identification parameters for columns in the somatic sensory cortex are the static properties of the neurons: the location of their receptive fields in the two dimensions of the body surface; the nature of the driving stimuli adequate to excite them, called the property of "modality"; and the rate of adaptation to a steady stimulus, a property determined at the level of the sensory receptor and thus one component of modality. These variables are set congruently by the segregated transsynaptic projection to the cerebral cortex of activity in small sets of first-order sensory fibers having common or closely overlapping receptive fields and a common sensory transducer capacity. They are mapped onto the X and Y dimensions of the postcentral somatic cortex, providing an example of an important general property of columnar organization: it allows the mapping of a number of variables within the two dimensions of the cerebral cortex.

Columnar organization for place and modality has now been observed in each of the topographical and cytoarchitectural divisions of the somatic sensory cortex, under a variety of experimental conditions and in several species: (1) in somatic area I of unanesthetized, neuromuscularly blocked squirrel and macaque monkeys (Werner and Whitsel, 1968; Mountcastle et al., 1969; Whitsel, Dryer, and Ropollo, 1971; Dryer et al., 1975); (2) in somatic I of waking, behaving macaque monkeys (Carli, LaMotte, and Mountcastle, 1971a, b); (3) in somatic area II in anesthetized cats (Carreras and Andersson, 1963) and unanesthetized, neuromuscularly blocked macaque monkeys (Whitsel, Petrucelli, and Werner, 1969); and (4) in anesthetized neonatal (Armstrong-James, 1975) and adult rats (Welker, 1971).

Werner, Whitsel, and their colleagues have made a major contribution to understanding the mapping of the body upon the somatic sensory cortex, and their results bear directly upon the nature of the columnar organization of this region (for review, see Werner and Whitsel, 1973). Each segment or small portion of a segment is mapped on the cortical surface into a long, narrow, sometimes sinuous strip extending anteroposteriorly across all of the cytoarchitectural areas (3a, 3b, 1, and 2) of the postcentral somatic cortex. These strips are arranged in such a way that movement along a particular mediolateral path on the cortex specifies movement along a continuous path on the body surface, formed by the sequential combination of movements across the individual dermatomes. Movement anteroposteriorly along any one of the dermatomal representations traces a path along the dermatome on the body surface. It has been known for a long time that the parameter of modality is also mapped differentially within this spatial representation. This mapping process generates an image of the body in cortical space that is topological in the sense that it preserves the connectivity of the body along specific paths without regard to the exact metric of the body itself. Orderly relations are maintained between ordered sets of elements in the space of the body and other ordered sets of elements in the representational space of the cortex, over afferent pathways some of which are divergent and recombinant.

The differential gradient for modality in the anteroposterior direction of a strip varies somewhat from one topographic region to another (for example, foot, leg, hand, arm, face) (Whitsel and Dryer, 1976), but in all regions there is a high probability that the columns of area 3a are specified by deep afferents including muscle afferents; those of area 3b by slowly adapting cutaneous afferents; those of area 1 by quickly adapting cutaneous afferents (Paul, Merzenich, and Goodman, 1972); and those of area 2 by deep afferents from joints, with some mixing in regions of transition. Further evidence is needed to clarify this general arrangement, for a major uncertainty remains: Are cortical columns of the somatic sensory cortex specified for place only in the mediolateral direction, or is there also a defining parameter in the anteroposterior direction along the narrow dermatomal representation? The latter seems more likely—that there is a necessary specification for place in both the X and the Y dimensions of the cortex and that modality is mapped congruently as a third static parameter.

Only preliminary studies have been made of the dynamics of neuronal processing in the columns of the somatic sensory cortex. There is evidence that activity in one column leads to inhibition of neurons in adjacent columns, whether of the same or of different modality specification (Mountcastle and Powell, 1959a, b). The mechanism of this inhibition is unknown. It is generated intracortically, perhaps via the putatively inhibitory interneuron described by Marin-Padilla (1970; see also Jones, 1975b). The terminals of these cells are distributed in thin, anteroposteriorly oriented, extended vertical discs. Such a distribution of inhibition is what would be required to isolate an active column or slab from its neighbors. It is likely that the inhibition imposed transsynaptically via the recurrent axon collaterals of the projection neurons of layers V and VI (Stephanis and Jasper, 1964) also plays a role in creating a pericolumnar inhibition.

Some neurons of the somatic sensory cortex are differentially sensitive to the direction of a stimulus moving across their peripheral receptive fields. This feature of the central representation of peripheral events first appears after two or more stages of intracortical processing, for Whitsel, Ropollo, and Werner (1972) discovered that cells displaying this dynamic property are preferentially located in layer III of the sensory cortex, with a smaller number in layer V. Directional selectivity appears to be a much more common property of cutaneous neurons of area 5 (Sakata et al., 1973; Mountcastle et al., 1975), to which many of the layer III pyramidal cells of the sensory cortex project. Although the evidence is so far only preliminary, these observations suggest that within a cutaneously specified column of the sensory cortex, there is preferential processing and integration, within a given channel leading to a particular output, of the neuronal events signaling stimulus attributes that are further elaborated in the projection target of that output channel.

Woolsey and Van der Loos (1970) discovered in the somatic sensory cortex of the rat a special anatomical arrangement that suggests u morphological basis for columnar organization in this area of this species. Each sinus hair of the contralateral face, and especially each of the mystacial vibrissae, is represented in a column of cells which, in layer IV, is clearly segregated into a "barrel" some 200–300 μm in diameter. The cell density in the wall of the barrel is 1.6 times that in its "hollow" center (Pasternak and Woolsey, 1975). Welker (1971) has shown by a single-neuron analysis that all the cells of a barrel, and the column of cells above and below it, are activated by movement of but a single contralateral vibrissa. Barrels are present also in the somatic sensory cortex of the mouse and of the Australian brush-tailed opossum, but they have not been found in any other of the large number of species examined (Feldman and Peters, 1974; Woolsey, Welker, and Schwartz, 1975).

In summary, the body form is mapped onto the postcentral somatic cortex of the primate with a preservation of topological order. Each small portion of the segmental innervation is projected to a long, sometimes sinuous, anteroposteriorly directed strip of cortex; strips vary in both A-P length and M-L width. Any single locus on the cortex is thus specified in its X and Y dimensions by the parameters of place. In addition, each column is further specified by the static parameter of modality. Thus the primary somatic sensory cortex illustrates several of the general characteristics of columnar organization:

1. Each local column is specified by the static parameters of place and modality, and rows of columns (or slabs) with the same dermatomal specification and those with the same modality specification are arranged more or less orthogonally to one another. There is preliminary evidence that other, more dynamic, variables are also mapped within this same two-dimensional matrix.

2. Its sets of columns are specifically linked to ordered sets of columns in other areas (see below).

3. This particular cortical area is dominated by its specific thalamocortical input, to such an extent that those regions in which sensory processing is thought to be most precise—the hand, foot, and face—are isolated from some corticocortical and callosal inputs.

4. The columnar organization is compatible with partially shifted overlap in the representation of the body form.

Evidence from Study of the Visual Cortex

It is in the visual cortex that we possess the most information and the strongest evidence for columnar organization, thanks largely to the elegant studies of Hubel and Wiesel, which they have recently summarized (1977). The mapping of visual space upon the striate cortex is determined by the distribution of geniculocortical fibers, while the segregation parameters for the columnar mapping of a number of variables are formed during the initial stages of intracortical processing. I wish to emphasize this point, for *the columnar processing units of the cortex appear to be specified both by their afferent inputs and by the nature of the intracortical processing of that input.* Hubel and Wiesel have shown by a combination of electrophysiological and a number of independent experimental anatomical methods that the columns of area 17 "form vertically disposed alternating left-eye and right-eye slabs, which in horizontal sections form alternating stripes about 400 μm thick, with occasional bifurcations and blind endings." Much narrower columns whose cells are selectively tuned to the orientation of short line segments are stacked in a direction more or less orthogonal to that of the ocular dominance stripes, so that each member of a local couplet of ocular dominance columns contains a complete 180° sequence of the slim orientation columns (or slabs). For any given neuron, the right-left dominance is determined by the afferent input, but the degree of that dominance and the property of orientation are determined by intracortical processes. Such a cross-matched combination of the binocular and orientation sets occupies an area of about 800 μm X 800 μm. I define such a set as a macrocolumn; it is a superimposed couplet of the ocular dominance and orientation hypercolumns defined by Hubel and Wiesel. Thus the visual cortex presents an example par excellence of how a number of variables can be mapped or represented in a two-dimensional matrix, by virtue of columnar organization. The two dimensions of the representation of space, the visual field, are mapped congruently with the variables of ocular dominance and orientation and undoubtedly still others as well (see below).

The compatibility of the principles of columnar organization and of partially shifted overlap is as clearly demonstrated in the visual as in the somatic sensory cortex. Here the aggregate receptive field of each macrocolumn overlaps by about one-half that of the adjacent sets, and the linear relation between magnification factor and receptive field size means that this overlap factor is invariant across the entire cortical representation of the visual field. Thus any oriented line segment presented in the visual field will be mapped maximally into a set of macrocolumns whose position is determined by the spatial location and linear extent of the stimulus. Within that selected set of macrocolumns, the locus of maximal activity will be determined by orientation. The partially shifted overlap of the representation of visual space determines that the row of maximally activated macrocolumns will be flanked on either side by sets less vigorously active, a lateral spread sharply limited by inhibition.

It is important to emphasize, as Hubel and Wiesel have done, the isolation of the processing function of the striate cortex. This area as a whole is the least interconnected of cortical regions. It sends and receives callosal fibers only along the representation of the vertical meridian and appears to receive no ipsilateral corticocortical connections. No U-fibers link any part of area 17 with any other part of that area, the tangential spread of the large majority of the intragrisial fibers is limited to about 1–2 mm (Fisken, Garey, and Powell, 1973), and there are good reasons to suppose that the principal function of the intragrisial fibers is the creation of lateral walls of inhibition that contribute to the dynamic isolation of an active column from its neighbors. Thus, while intracortical processing within area 17 is an essential step leading to visual perception, it is probably correct to say that visual perception does not "occur" there, but rather within a series of complex distributed systems in each of which a locus in area 17 is an integral part. For the most complex aspects of vision, a primate possessing only area 17 among all visual and visual associative cortical areas would probably be perceptually blind.

Studies of the dynamic activity of visual cortical neurons suggest that within any given macrocolumn, processing for different stimulus attributes proceeds along parallel channels. The general rule seems to be that the attributes selected in a given pathway leading to an output channel are those further elaborated in the target area of the channel: the processing and distribution functions of a cortical column are then combined. This principle is shown, for example, by the recent findings of Poggio and his colleagues, who have studied the dynamic processing of neural activity in the foveal visual cortex of waking monkeys trained to fixate steadily on a target even though a variety of other visual stimuli are presented (Poggio, Doty, and Talbot, 1977; Poggio and Fisher, 1977). Poggio has measured the spatial-frequency tuning properties of striate neurons, their sensitivity to moving gratings, and certain aspects of binocular interaction including disparity sensitivity. As regards spatial-frequency sensitivity, the majority of cells of the deep layers of the cortex have the properties of "movement analyzers," appropriate for the brain stem oculomotor control system upon which many neurons of the infragranular layers project. In contrast, neurons of the supragranular layers appear to function as "form analyzers," to a certain degree independently of movement. The output trajectory from these layers is largely to areas 18 and 19, where it is likely that further processing leads eventually to the perception of spatial structure. Thus different sets of output neurons possess common static properties of locus of receptive field, ocularity, and orientation, but the channels leading to them accentuate and elaborate different dynamic properties of the input signals.

It has been known for some time that many neurons of the cat's visual areas (Barlow, Blakemore, and Pettigrew, 1967; Nikara, Bishop, and Pettigrew, 1968; Pettigrew, Nikara, and Bishop, 1968) and in area 18 of the monkey cortex (Hubel and Wiesel, 1970) display receptive field disparity. It has been suggested that these neurons may therefore play a role in the central neural mechanisms in stereopsis. Poggio and Fisher (1977) have recently identified neurons with such receptive field disparities in area 17 of the waking, behaving monkey. They observed depth-tuned excitatory and inhibitory neurons that, in addition to playing a candidate role in the neural mechanisms for stereopsis, may serve to maintain visual fixation. These tuned neurons were found throughout the cortical layers, but in greatest proportion in the lower layers that project subcortically. By contrast, other neurons sensitive to a larger range of disparities either in front of ("near neurons") or behind ("far neurons") the plane of fixation are more plentiful in the supragranular layers. Cells of these layers (II and III) are known to project to other cortical regions, mainly 18 and 19, where it is believed the neural mechanisms for stereoscopic vision are further elaborated. These neurons may also contribute to the cortical control of oculomotor vergence leading to fusion.

This general idea has received further support from the combined electrophysiological and anatomical studies of Zeki, who has explored a set of projection zones of area 17 in areas 18 and 19 and in the cortex of the posterior bank of the superior temporal sulcus in the monkey. In each of these zones he has observed a further elaboration of the processing of a particular stimulus attribute (Zeki, 1974, 1975, 1977).

In summary, the striate visual cortex illustrates several of the general properties of columnar organization:

1. Several variables are mapped within its two-dimensional matrix.

2. Its macrocolumns function as input-output processing devices such that parallel processing within each allows the selection of certain dynamic stimulus attributes for elaboration along restricted channels leading to particular outputs (commonly those attributes are accentuated in the processing mechanisms of the target regions).

3. Its sets of columns are specifically linked to ordered sets of columns in other cortical areas and in modules of subcortical structures upon which it projects.

4. The visual cortex of the monkey is dominated by its geniculostriate projection and thus resembles the hand and foot areas of the somatic sensory cortex in the degree of input isolation.

5. The columnar organization of the visual cortex is compatible with the principle of partially shifted overlap in the representation of the visual fields in neural space.

Evidence from Study of the Auditory Cortex

It has been known for a long time that the cochlear partition, and thus the frequency of stimulating sounds, is represented in the

"primary" auditory cortex A-1 in an orderly fashion, a body of knowledge due in large part to the extensive series of evoked-potential experiments carried out by Woolsey and his colleagues (for review, see Woolsey,
1960). Similar methods have been used to identify the auditory cortex
of in the human brain on the superior surface of the temporal lobe in
an area corresponding to the transverse temporal gyri (Celesia, 1976).
The koniocortex of this region is the most markedly columniated of
any heterotypical cortex; its radial arrangement of cells is obvious in
sections cut normal to the cortical surface. Indeed, Sousa-Pinta (1973)
has described in the cat's A-1 vertical cylinders of cells in the middle
layers with diameters of 50–60 μm and with cell-poor centers. Studies
of the physiological properties of single neurons of A-1 have revealed
that cells encountered as a microelectrode passes down such a vertical
column are tuned to a nearly identical frequency and that their tuning
curves have sharp roll-offs in both directions, due at least in part to
lateral inhibition (Parker, 1965; Abeles and Goldstein, 1970; Merzenich
and Brugge, 1973; Merzenich, Knight, and Roth, 1975; Imig and
Adrian, 1977). A similar columnar organization for best frequency has
been established for the anterior auditory area as well (Knight, 1977).
The overlap of the tuning curves of neurons in adjacent isofrequency
strips is sufficient to account for the partially shifted overlap of frequency representation observed in surface-mapping experiments.

It was Tunturi who first suggested that other properties of
auditory signals might be mapped along each isofrequency contour or
strip of the cortex, in a direction orthogonal to that of the change in
frequency (Tunturi, 1952; Tunturi and Dudman, 1958). This has now
been shown to be the case in the cat by the important new study of
Imig and Adrian (1977), and in the monkey by the initial studies of
Brugge and Merzenich (1973). In the high-frequency region of the cat's
A-1, aural dominance and binaural interaction are the properties that
vary along the long dimension of an isofrequency band. Neurons
located along the perpendicular axis of the cortex, within such a band,
display similar properties of frequency sensitivity and binaural interaction. Slanting penetrations within an isofrequency band often pass from
a zone in which neurons exhibit one kind of binaural interaction to one
in which they exhibit another.

Binaural stimulation may produce a suppression of response, as
compared with the response to monaural stimulation, and in all such
cases the contralateral ear is dominant. On the other hand, binaural
stimulation may produce summation, and in this case either ear may

dominate. The suppression and summation columns are arranged in continuous bands placed more or less orthogonally to the isofrequency contours. Within each summation set there is a further columniation for which the identification parameter is ear dominance. It is well known that the interaural intensity difference provides the cue for localization in space of high-frequency sounds (that is, sounds above about 3,000 Hz).

Studies of the auditory cortex of the monkey are much less advanced than those in the cat, but it is already clear that the representation of frequency in A-1 of the monkey is also in terms of isofrequency contours or bands located at right angles to the line of representation of the cochlear partition. These isofrequency bands extend throughout the cellular layers of the cortex, in accord with columnar organization (Brugge and Merzenich, 1973). One observation made by these investigators is of great interest in the present context. They observed in the bands for frequencies of 2,500 Hz and below that neurons in columns were most sensitive to the interaural delay. It is this property of interaural stimulus delay that accounts for the capacity to locate sound of low frequency in surrounding space.

Suga (1977) has discovered in the auditory cortex of the mustacho bat an example of columnar organization that illustrates the advantage conferred by the freedom to map a number of variables in two dimensions. This animal emits orientation sounds with a long constant-frequency (CF) component followed by a short frequency-modulated (FM) component. The CF component is used for target detection and measurement of target velocity, with Doppler-shifted compensation. The FM component is used for localization and ranging of the target. The most intense part of the CF is the second harmonic at about 61 kHz, which sweeps down to 51 kHz during the last few msec of the signal. About 30% of the primary auditory cortex is devoted to columns that are closely specified for the CF component in the second harmonic of the orientation sounds and its Doppler-shifted echoes. Columns are specified along radial and concentric axes for the two identification parameters of frequency and amplitude, and this representation occupies a disproportionately large share of the auditory cortex.

In summary, the primary auditory cortex is organized in a columnar manner, and although the evidence is still incomplete, the identification parameters in the X and Y dimensions suggest that two intersecting bands of columns map sound frequency against the neural transforms of those stimulus attributes necessary for localizing sounds in space. These are the interaural intensity differences for high frequencies and interaural time differences for low frequencies (below 2,500 Hz). More evidence will be needed to establish this general model with certainty, and undoubtedly other dynamic parameters are also mapped along the axis of the isofrequency bands of columns, but the general similarity to the arrangements in the visual and somatic sensory cortices is obvious.

Evidence from Study of the Precentral Motor Cortex

The precentral motor cortex was until recently the most intensively studied but least understood of the heterotypical areas of the neocortex. Significant advances in understanding the functional organization of this region and its role in the control of movement have been made in the last decade by the application of new methods. Notable among these are the recording of the electrical signs of the activity of single neurons in the motor cortex of waking monkeys trained to emit repetitively a defined movement (Evarts, 1975), intracortical stimulation and recording through a penetrating microelectrode (Asanuma, 1973, 1975), and several new methods for tracing projections to and from such a cortical region. I call attention to only a small part of the large literature that has resulted, in particular that dealing with the functional organization of the precentral motor cortex.

Asanuma and his colleagues have used the method of intracortical microstimulation to produce convincing evidence that those loci within the cortex at which stimulation with weak currents (4 μa) produces small movements of a distal joint, often executed by a single muscle, are arrayed in vertical columns 0.5–1.0 mm in diameter, which match the radial cell columns so characteristic of this area (Asanuma and Rosen, 1972a,b). They were also able by recording through the stimulating microelectrode to define the afferent input to the motor cortical cells in the immediate vicinity. These cells were commonly activated by stimulation of receptors in deep tissues in and about the joint moved by the local intracortical stimulation. Only those columns in which stimulation produced movement of the fingers contained neurons with cutaneous receptive fields. These commonly lay on the glabrous skin of the hand in such locations as to be activated by the movement evoked by local stimulation. The input-output loop thus composed is thought to play a role in tactually guided movement of the hand and fingers and in instinctive grasping. These observations have been confirmed in principle by a number of investigators (Doetsch and Gardner, 1972; Lenon and Porter, 1976). Others have emphasized the more distributed nature of the "colonies" of pyramidal tract neurons related to a particular muscle (Phillips, 1969; Anderssen et al., 1975). A significant finding by Jankowska, Padel, and Tanaka (1975a,b) was that although the excited loci for a given muscle were more widely distributed than suggested by the observations of Asanuma, they were discontinuous. Thus one working hypothesis concerning the functional organization of the motor cortex is that radial columns of neurons processing input to output directed at a single motoneuron pool are clustered together, with an overlap where the thinning edge of a cluster meets the edges of clusters of columns related to other muscles. According to this idea there is complete compatibility between the columnar organization of the motor cortex and the partially shifted overlap emphasized by Phillips (1969) and others. One might suppose that the motor cortical patterns controlling movement result from the dynamic combination into continually forming and dissolving sets of active columns related to one, two, or many muscles involved in a particular phase of ongoing movement. The organizing commands for the composition of these *movement sets* are envisaged to arise elsewhere rather than in the precentral motor cortex per se. Thus the old and oft-repeated question, "Does the motor cortex think in terms of movements or muscles?" appears redundant. The motor cortex is an intermediate level in the true Jacksonian sense: it does not "think" and both movements and muscles are "represented" within it, though each in a different way.

Asanuma and Rosen (1973) have elucidated still further the columnar organization in the motor cortex by using two penetrating microelectrodes, one for stimulation and the other for recording. Stimulation in the upper layers was found to elicit excitation locally and in the lower layers as well, in a column slightly less than 1 mm in diameter; that same stimulation produced a pericolumnar zone of inhibition. Stimulation in the deeper layers produced local excitation, and the same pericolumnar inhibition, perhaps identical in mechanism to that described by Stephanis and Jasper (1964) as being caused by impulses in the recurrent axon collaterals of the cells of origin of pyramidal tract fibers. Surprisingly, no excitation of neurons in the supragranular layers was produced by stimulation in the deep layers.

In summary, the motor cortex is organized into cell columns about 1 mm in diameter, but the shape and geometry of the columns or strips is unknown. The groups of columns related to particular seg-

mental interneuron and motoneuron pools appear in clusters, with overlap at their edges with adjacent clusters devoted to other muscles. The
mapping parameter in the X and Y dimensions appears to be location in
the pattern of the body musculature. One might predict that other,
more dynamic aspects of the pattern of neuronal activity are mapped
into these same X and Y dimensions, perhaps by a further columniation
within the larger columns so far defined only in topographic terms. A
dynamic pericolumnar inhibition appears to be exerted both by intra-
grisially projecting axons and by the action of recurrent collaterals of
projection neurons of the infragranular layers.

Evidence from Study of the Parietal Homotypical Cortex

The homotypical cortex of the parietal lobe of the monkey
exhibits the vertical cording of neurons and the functional characteristics of columnar organization (Mountcastle et al., 1975; Lynch et al.,
1977). These regions differ remarkably from the heterotypical areas
considered hitherto, for they are neither dominated by a single afferent input, as are the primary sensory areas, nor linked unconditionally
to peripheral effectors, as in the motor cortex. The specifying parameters for columnar sets in the homotypical parietal cortex must be
sought in experiments in which electrophysiological observations can be
made in animals trained to emit a series of behavioral acts—acts chosen
because evidence obtained on other grounds suggests their relevance to
the region under study. The columnar sets of areas 5 and 7, when
studied in this way, all appear to have one common specifying characteristic: their cells are active in relation to the animal's action upon and
within his immediately surrounding environment and also to the spatial
relations between his body and its parts, the gravitational field, and that
environment (Mountcastle, 1975, 1976, 1977). Within area 7 there are
different sets of columns whose cells are active during (1) projection of
the arm toward an object of interest; (2) manipulation of an object;
(3) fixation of gaze and thus of visual attention; (4) visually evoked but
not spontaneous saccadic movement of the eyes; (5) slow pursuit tracking movement of the eyes; and (6) the sudden appearance of objects in
the periphery of the visual field (these are the only neurons so far identified in the parietal cortex that are "visual" in the usual sense). The
columnar segregation of these groups of cells with quite different properties is shown by the facts that (1) microelectrode penetrations normal
to the cortical surface and along the vertically arranged cell columns

have a high probability of encountering cells of only one class, and (2) penetrations that pass in directions slanting across the cell columns traverse blocks of tissue within which cells are all of one type or another rather than intermingled. So far little is known about the exact size or shape of the columns in the parietal cortex or about the dynamics of neuronal processing within them.

It is my proposition that each of these classes of columnar sets of the parietal cortex is related by specific extrinsic connections to similarly segregated sets of modules in other cortical regions and in subcortical nuclei as well, and that these closely interconnected modular sets of different large brain entities form precisely connected, distributed systems, serving distributed functions.

A Central Core System Projecting to the Neocortex, without Columnar Organization

The general concept of columnar organization does not preclude the possibility that other systems may engage the cortex in different ways, particularly those involved in general regulatory functions rather than detailed information processing. One example is the noradrenergic system that arises in the locus coeruleus and projects to very widely distributed portions of the central nervous system, including the entire neocortex (for review, see Moore and Bloom, 1977). This direct neocortical projection system has been demonstrated in a number of species, including primates. The locus coeruleus emits two identifiable ascending tracts that reach the neocortex directly. They pass upward through the subthalamus; the medial component reaches the neocortex via the cingulum bundle, the lateral via the external capsule. The special aspect of this system is that from the two local points of entry, fibers pass tangentially to reach every cortical region and every cortical layer. Molliver and his colleagues (1977) have used an immunohistochemical method to trace this system in detail, and in their montage reconstructions the neocortex is seen to be interlaced in all directions by a web of fine noradrenergic fibers at 30–40 μm intervals. Each layer except IV contains radial, tangential, or oblique axons arranged in such a manner that any individual noradrenergic axon may influence adjacent cortical columns over very long distances. It appears that any single cell of the locus coeruleus may project very widely upon the brain, including large areas of the neocortex, and sustain an immense and divergent axonal field. The exact mode of termination of these fibers is still uncertain and may include both traditional synaptic terminations and transmitter release sites *en passage,* but it is obvious that the system has the capacity to influence directly every cell in the neocortex.

The functional significance of this system is equally uncertain. One may conjecture from its distribution that it exerts a controlling or regulating influence upon the neocortex and that this might occur by direct synaptic engagement, by release of synaptic transmitter agents "at a distance," by both of these means, or by regulation of blood flow and vascular permeability (Raichle et al., 1975). The role this system is known to play in sleep mechanisms may be only the most obvious of these controls. Whatever the nature of its influence upon the cortex—which may even include its maturation—there is no sign of "columnar organization" in the way it engages the neocortex.

Intrinsic Organization of the Neocortex

An understanding of the functional organization of the neocortical module requires a flow diagram of the structural linkages between its inputs and its outputs. It is not yet possible to construct such a diagram, though recent studies have provided many of the facts it will require, as regards both intrinsic and extrinsic connectivity. Szentágothai has summarized this growing body of information in a series of successively more complete models which have been of considerable heuristic value (Szentágothai, 1973, 1975, 1976; see also Garey, 1976, and Colonnier, 1966, 1968).

The general plan is as follows. Afferent fibers that reach the neocortex come from three major sources: from specifically related nuclei of the dorsal thalamus; from other cortical areas of the same hemisphere; and via the corpus callosum from usually homologous but sometimes heterologous areas of the contralateral hemisphere. Less dense and more diffusely distributed innervations arise in the generalized thalamic nuclei, the basilar forebrain regions, and certain monaminergic nuclei of the brain stem. The terminals of extrinsic afferents to the cortex are always of the excitatory type (asymmetrical profiles with round vesicles) (Garey and Powell, 1971; Jones and Powell, 1970), but they make up a relatively small portion of all excitatory terminals in the cortex: estimates vary from 5% to 20%. The major classes of corticofugal axons are ipsilateral corticocortical, commissural corticocortical, corticothalamic, and a large class whose targets include, in different combinations for different areas, the basal ganglia, mesencephalon, pons, medulla, and spinal cord. Afferent systems of different origin engage different but overlapping laminar targets within the cortex. The densest concentration of terminals of specific thalamocortical fibers is in layers IV and III-B (Jones and Powell, 1970; Hubel and Wiesel, 1972; Sloper, 1973; Jones, 1975a; Winfield and Powell, 1976; Jones and Burton, 1976). Those of the generalized thalamocortical system and those of brain stem origin terminate in all layers, but especially in layer I. Ipsilateral corticocortical and commissural fibers terminate predominantly in the supragranular layers, most densely in layers III and IV (see, for example, Jones, Burton, and Porter, 1975; Goldman and Nauta, 1977).

There are only rare exceptions to the general rules that all the pyramidal cells of the cortex emit extrinsically directed axons, that all extrinsic axons arising in the cortex come from pyramidal cells, and that all extrinsic axons are excitatory in synaptic action. The pyramidal cells of origin of different efferent systems are precisely segregated by layer. The cell bodies of corticothalamic fibers are located in layer VI (Lund et al., 1975; Gilbert and Kelly, 1975; Jones and Wise, 1977); those of the corticocortical systems in layer III (Shoumura, 1974; Shoumura, Ando, and Kato, 1975; Lund et al., 1975; Jones, Burton, and Porter, 1975; Jones and Wise, 1977; Glickstein and Whitteridge, 1976); and those of other descending systems to the basal ganglia, brain stem, and spinal cord in layer V (Berrevoets and Kuypers, 1975; Humphrey and Rietz, 1976; Jones et al., 1977; Jones and Wise, 1977).

There is evidence that some (unknown) proportion of the excitatory terminals of extrinsic afferents end monosynaptically upon the spiny processes of pyramidal cells, thus providing a monosynaptic "throughput" pathway. However, it is likely that the large majority of extrinsic afferents end upon the local interneurons of the cortex, the heterogeneous class of stellate cells. These interneurons vary in location, size, sign of synaptic action, extent and type of dendritic field, and axonal ramification. They have been classified in a number of ways (Lund, 1973; Jones, 1975b). It is likely that the spiny stellate cell of layers IV and III-B is a major target of the specific thalamocortical fibers. This cell is excitatory in synaptic action, and its terminals make powerful cascading synapses upon the spines of the apical dendrites of pyramidal cells (LeVay, 1973; Lund, 1973; Lund and Boothe, 1975; Jones, 1975a). Other interneurons are also excitatory and receive direct extrinsic input; together they must provide a system of echeloned pathways in both series and parallel configuration from input to out-put, undoubtedly encased by powerful feedback and feedforward loops as well. The pattern of distribution of the excitatory stellate inter-neurons in the neocortex is one of very dense and powerful synaptic connectivity to the output cells in the vertical direction across the cor-tical layers and rapidly thinning connectivity in the horizontal direc-tion. One particular type of inhibitory interneuron, the large basket cell of layers III, IV, and V, emits an axonal distribution field arranged in a narrow, elongated vertical disc within which the individual axonal terminals clasp in basketlike arrangements the cell bodies of the pyrami-dal cells within that field (Marin-Padilla, 1969, 1970). This class of cells is likely to exert a strong synaptic pericolumnar inhibition. Other, smaller inhibitory basket cells are thought to isolate smaller cylinders of space within the larger column. The total number of inhibitory termi-nals (symmetrical profiles with flattened or multiform vesicles) in the cortex is small compared with the number of excitatory ones, but they are strategically placed upon the somata and proximal dendrites of pyramidal cells, so that their suppressive effects per synaptic event can be very powerful.

Almost all extrinsic axons emit recurrent collaterals that branch repeatedly in a spherelike domain up to 3 mm in diameter about the cell of origin, penetrating all the cellular layers from the place of recur-rence, usually in layer VI. The exact terminations of the branches of these recurrent axons is not clear, but undoubtedly some emit axonal terminals to the spiny processes of the dendrites of adjacent pyramidal cells and are thus excitatory to them. However, it is likely that the large majority of the terminal branches of these axonal collaterals terminate upon inhibitory interneurons. This is suggested by the fact that the transsynaptic action of an antidromic impulse in an extrinsic axon, upon neighboring pyramidal cells, is a small and transient depolariza-tion followed by a very large and prolonged hyperpolarization. The net result is a powerful inhibition (Stephanis and Jasper, 1964). The distri-bution pattern of the recurrent axonal collateral system suggests that intense activity in any small group of output cells will exert a powerful pericolumnar inhibition. Thus the cortical column is established by virtue of anatomical connections—its specific afferent input and its ver-tically oriented intrinsic connectivity—but also in a dynamic manner by a strong pericolumnar inhibition exerted by the large basket cell inter-neurons and the pyramidal cell axonal collaterals. It is this dynamic isolation which makes the concept of columnar organization compatible with that of partially shifted overlap.

It should be emphasized that the complexities of the neuronal processing mechanisms in the neocortex are not limited by classical synaptic connectivity. Recent studies have shown that in many places in the nervous system, including the neocortex, dendrites may themselves be presynaptic to other dendrites, or even to axon terminals. These elements are frequently arranged in "triads," which appear to be local processing units that may by their integrated outputs affect events in the neuronal elements of larger circuits (Schmitt, Dev, and Smith, 1976). Finally, a number of what are regarded as general regulatory systems engage the cortex in all its layers. It is presently surmised that these systems play a level-setting role, but it is possible that they exert a more focused and differential action upon cortical neuronal excitability.

Extrinsic Connectivity of the Neocortex

A major advance of the last two decades has been the discovery of a much more detailed and specific connectivity between brain parts than had hitherto been supposed. New methods for light microscopy, particularly the reduced silver methods for staining degenerating axon terminals, led to a series of important discoveries by a number of investigators. More recently, advantage has been taken of the axoplasmic transport of identifiable molecules to trace connections in both anterograde and retrograde directions. The labeling of transmitter agents or their synthesizing enzymes for fluorescent or immunofluorescent microscopy has made it possible to trace even the finest axons to their terminations.

The mass of information now available concerning neocortical connectivity cannot be summarized briefly, but certain general principles begin to emerge. Each neocortical region receives (is defined by) a projection from a dorsal thalamic nucleus and projects back to that nucleus in closely ordered registry. All neocortical regions receive, in addition, afferent inflows from a number of generalized regulating systems: from the basilar forebrain regions, from the generalized nuclei of the dorsal thalamus, and from certain monaminergic nuclei of the brain stem. Generally, homologous neocortical areas of the two hemispheres are reciprocally linked via the great commissures of the forebrain, but there are two known exceptions: the striate cortex (except for the region in which the vertical meridian is represented) and certain parts of the somatic sensory cortex have no commissural connections at all. Uncommonly, a cortical region is linked to heterologous as well as to homologous contralateral areas. Within a single hemisphere there is a step-by-step outward progression of corticocortical connections from primary sensory areas onto successively adjacent areas of the homotypical cortex of the parietal, occipital, and temporal lobes, and each of the successive "higher-order" convergent regions is reciprocally linked with more anterior areas of the frontal lobe. Those receiving the most highly convergent projections are linked via two-way connections with areas of the limbic lobe. There are, however, many exceptions to this general scheme.

On the output side, the neocortex as a whole projects upon almost every other major entity of the nervous system: the basal ganglia, dorsal thalamus, mesencephalon, brain stem, and spinal cord, but the number and the patterns of their efferent projections differ greatly from one region to another. Many of them form massive reentrant systems, for example, the reciprocal systems linking dorsal thalamus and neocortex, or the large reentrant components converging upon the motor cortex from the basal ganglia and cerebellum, or the descending projections linked to brain stem relay nuclei of the auditory and somatic systems. These systems have many points of entry and exit. They should not be regarded as closed, reverberating circuits.

The number of extrinsic connections identified for single cytoarchitectural areas of the neocortex is much larger than had once been thought. Even the striate cortex, the least interconnected of those neocortical regions that have been studied intensively, is linked by fiber systems to and from at least 10 separate structures. Area 7 of the parietal lobe entertains 17 such connections, and area 3b of the postcentral somatic sensory cortex has connections with no fewer than 29 different targets/sources! Is it possible that each modular unit of a cytoarchitecturally defined area makes all the connections that have been identified for that area? Discoveries of the last two years suggest that this is not the case. Grant, Landgren, and Silvenius (1975) found that small lesions made in area 3a of the cat neocortex produce antegrade degeneration of terminals in restricted zones of areas 2, 3b, and 4. These zones are arranged in a columnar manner, each column is about 1 mm in diameter, and the columns are interspersed with zones of the same cytoarchitectural area free of any degeneration. Shanks, Rockel, and Powell (1975) and Jones, Burton, and Porter (1975) discovered independently that the terminals of commissural fibers linking the somatic sensory areas of the monkey are arranged in columns that cluster in mediolateral bands or groups at the transitional zones between the several cytoarchitectural areas of the postcentral gyrus, separated by columnar zones free of any terminals. Moreover, the cells of origin of these commissural fibers, which lie in layer III-B, were found to be clustered in groups, as if located in some columns but not in others. The columns that send and receive commissural fibers appear to be the same. Corticocortical fibers reaching the postcentral from the precentral gyrus also terminate in isolated clusters, but whether those columns sending and receiving ipsilateral association fibers are identical with those sending and receiving commissural fibers is not known. Shanks, Pearson, and Powell (1977) also found that the intrinsic fiber connections of the monkey's postcentral gyrus terminate in bands or clusters that appear to be coincident with those linking the two postcentral gyri via the corpus callosum. Kunzle (1976) showed a similar alternating arrangement of vertically oriented zones that did and did not send and receive the commissural fibers linking areas 4 and 6 with homologous areas of the contralateral hemisphere.

Goldman and Nauta (1976a, 1977) found that both commissural and ipsilateral association fibers arising in the frontal granular cortex terminate within their diverse cortical targets in vertically oriented columns, 200–500 μm wide, which alternate in regular sequence with zones of comparable width that are free of such terminals. In a nearly reciprocal experiment, Jacobsen and Trojanowski (1977) found that the cells of origin of the commissural fibers arising in the frontal granular cortex of the monkey are located in clusters, alternating with zones free of such cells, a finding consonant with a vertical mode of organization. Goldman and Nauta (1976b) also made the important observation that the segregation of the zones of distribution of cortical efferents is not confined to cortical targets, for the terminals of axons projecting from the frontal granular cortex to the caudate nucleus, in the monkey, are segregated into clusters separated by zones free of such terminals. This finding has been confirmed by Jones et al. (1977).

These new experimental findings suggest that columniation of the intracortical terminal distributions of afferent fibers and of the cells that emit them is a common feature of neocortical organization, just as is the pattern of termination of thalamocortical afferents (Hubel and Wiesel, 1972). Moreover, it appears likely that the total set of columns composing a cytoarchitectural area is fractionated into subsets, each of which sends and receives a particular fraction of the total set of connections of the area. It is not likely that any one subset of columns has no extrinsic connections at all or that any other set entertains them all. A further specification of subset connections is obviously a major objective of present anatomical research.

General Statements

The Modular Construction of the Nervous System

The general proposition is that the large entities of the nervous system which we know as the dorsal horn, reticular formation, dorsal thalamus, basal ganglia, neocortex, and so forth, are themselves composed of local circuits. These circuits form modules which vary from place to place in cell number, structural organization, or mode of neuronal processing, but which are at the first level of analysis similar within any single large entity. Modules are grouped into entities by virtue of a dominant extrinsic connection, the need to replicate a common function over a topographic field, or certain intermodular interactions. All the elements in the set of modules composing an entity may not be linked to all of its extrinsic connections; thus the total set of modules composing an entity is fractionated into subsets by different linkages to similarly segregated subsets in other large entities. These specific connections may preserve neighborhood relations in the topographic sense and in any case preserve topologic order. The closely linked subsets of several different large entities thus form precisely connected, distributed systems; these distributed systems are conceived as serving distributed functions.

The Columnar Organization of the Neocortex: The Basic Unit

The basic unit of operation in the neocortex is a vertically arranged group of cells heavily interconnected in the vertical axis running across the cortical layers and sparsely connected horizontally. This idea originated as a prediction made from anatomical studies of intracortical cellular arrangements and received its strongest support from the results of electrophysiological studies of the primary sensory areas of the neocortex. More recently, additional evidence supporting this hypothesis has come from a large number of studies of both intrinsic and extrinsic cortical connectivity, particularly from those in which new methods have been used to identify the cells of origin and the locus of termination of connecting axons.

I define the basic modular unit of the neocortex as a minicolumn. It is a vertically oriented cord of cells formed by the migration of neurons from the germinal epithelium of the neural tube along the radial glial cells to their destined locations in the cortex, as described by Rakic. If this minicolumn is comparable in size to the cortical cylinders in which Rockel, Hiorns, and Powell (1974) made neuronal counts, it contains about 110 cells. This figure is almost invariant between different neocortical areas and different species of mammals, except for the striate cortex of primates, where it is 260. Such a cord of cells occupies a gently curving, nearly vertical cylinder of cortical space with a diameter of about 30 μm. The total volume of the human neocortex is about 1,000 cm^3. Assuming an average thickness of 2,500 μm, the neocortex of the human brain has a surface area of about 4,000 cm^2 and contains about 600 million minicolumns and on the order of 50 billion neurons.

The Large Processing Unit of the Neocortex: Many-Variable Mapping in a Package of Minicolumns

Studies of the primary sensory and motor cortices and of two areas of the homotypical cortex of the parietal lobe have revealed that it is possible to identify within the neocortex a much larger processing unit than the minicolumn. The diameters or widths of this larger unit have been given as 500 μm to 1,000 μm for different areas. Moreover, it is clear that this larger processing unit may vary in its cross-sectional form, being round, or oval, or slablike in shape. Given the dimensions of the larger processing unit of the visual cortex, the macrocolumn as I have defined it, one can estimate that the human neocortex contains about 600,000 of these larger processing units, each packaging several hundred minicolumns. The calculations have a high degree of uncertainty and are given to indicate order of magnitude only.

The larger processing unit has been defined in terms of both the static and dynamic properties of its neurons. For the visual cortex, place on the visual cortex is of course in the first instance defined by place in the visual field. The larger processing unit is defined by ocularity and by orientation. The latter property results from intracortical processing and is specified by afferent input only in the topographical sense. In the somatic sensory cortex place on the body surface and modality type are the initial defining parameters, but it is still uncertain whether two dimensions are needed for the designation of place; if so, modality would then become a third defining parameter, mapped congruently. For the auditory cortex, sound frequency and those aspects of binaural interaction that define the location of a sound in space are the defining parameters. Further, it appears that within the domain of these larger processing units, other variables, particularly those of a dynamic nature, can be mapped onto the X and Y dimensions of the cortex, with no disturbance of topological relations. I propose that this "submapping" is ordered in terms of sets of minicolumns, and in the limit in terms of single ones. On this hypothesis the minicolumn is regarded as the irreducibly small processing unit of the neocortex. It may be, for example, that the minicolumn is the mapping unit for the parameter of orientation specificity within each ocular-dominant half of the couplet composing the macrocolumn of the striate cortex. A similar example is suggested by the mediolateral mapping for aural dominance and the various forms of binaural interaction observed along the isofrequency bands of the auditory cortex.

The property of many-variable representation is a salient feature of an organization in terms of vertical units and one of its important characteristics in terms of cortical function. A series of trade-offs must exist between the degree of fine-grainedness of a topographic representation and the number of variables mapped to it. In the somatic sensory or visual cortex, for example, the specificity required for the representation of place may limit markedly the number of variables simultaneously mapped to the regions. In those homotypical areas of neocortex where topography is much less precise or indeed absent altogether, a large number of variables can be mapped through a given area with preservation of ordered relations between sets on the source side, those within the area, and those in target structures. That is, a number of distributed systems can be mapped through a given area of cortex, thus allowing an integration of their activities (their functions) with properties of that area determined by some other input to it.

A cortical column is a complex processing and distributing unit that links a number of inputs to several outputs. The cells of origin of different output pathways appear to be sharply segregated by cortical layer. Although the intracolumnar channels making these links must certainly overlap and interact, there is evidence that the nature of neuronal processing may differ in different channels. Poggio and his colleagues have given examples of this phenomenon from their work on the visual cortex in waking monkeys. They found that the dynamic properties of spatial-frequency tuning, movement sensitivity, and fine and gross stereopsis are differentially emphasized in the different output channels. It appears likely that other pathways from input to output may be very short, even monosynaptic. Such "throughputs" emphasize the distribution function of a cortical column, as if certain aspects of input signals were being quickly routed to output targets for further processing.

An important property of the intracortical processing mechanisms is what I have termed *pericolumnar inhibition*. It is a powerful mechanism for the functional isolation of active columns from their neighbors, one that brings the concept of columnar organization into conformity with that of partially shifted overlap. The latter is the general principle that as a stimulus of restricted size is shifted in small steps across a receptor sheet, it brings to action a series of shifted but overlapping populations of cortical elements. Pericolumnar inhibition will tend to limit very sharply the lateral spread of activity around the columnar sets most strongly activated by such a local stimulus. This principle undoubtedly holds also for areas of the cortex other than sensory.

Functional Properties of Distributed Systems

It is well known from classical neuroanatomy that many of the large entities of the brain are interconnected by extrinsic pathways into complex systems, including massive reentrant circuits. Three sets of recent discoveries, described above, have put the systematic organization of the brain in a new light. The first is that many of the major structures of the brain are constructed by replication of identical multicellular units. These modules are local neural circuits of hundreds or thousands of cells linked together by a complex intramodular connectivity. The modules of any one entity are more or less similar throughout, but those of different entities may differ strikingly. The modular unit of the neocortex is the vertically organized group of cells I have described earlier. These basic units are single translaminar cords of neurons, the minicolumns, which in some areas are packaged into larger processing units whose size and form appear to differ from one place to another. Nevertheless, the qualitative nature of the processing function of the neocortex is thought to be similar in different areas, though that intrinsic processing apparatus may be subject to modification as a result of past history, particularly during critical periods in ontogenetic development.

The second important factor leading to a change in concepts concerning brain function is the accumulation of a vast amount of information concerning the extrinsic connectivity between large entities of the brain. These links are now known to be far more numerous, selective, and specific than previously supposed. The third fact of importance is the discovery that each one of the modules of a large entity does not entertain all the connections known for the entity. Thus the total set of modules of a large entity is fractionated into subsets, each linked by a particular pattern of connections to similarly segregated subsets in other large entities. The linked sets of modules of the several entities are defined as a distributed system. It is obvious that the total number of distributed systems within the brain is much larger than had once been thought, and perhaps by several orders of magnitude. Thus major entities are parts of many distributed systems, contributing to each a property determined for the entity by those connections common to all of its modular subsets and by the particular quality of their intrinsic processing. Even a single module of such an entity may be a member of several (though not many) distributed systems.

Distributed systems are thus composed of large numbers of modular elements linked together in echeloned parallel and serial arrangements. Information flow through such a system may follow a number of different pathways, and the dominance of one path or another is a dynamic and changing property of the system. Such a system has many entries and exits and has access to outflow systems of the brain at many levels. A distributed system displays a redundancy of potential loci of command, and the command function may from time to time reside in different loci of the system, in particular in that part possessing the most urgent and necessary information.

An important feature of such distributed systems, particularly those central to primary sensory and motor systems, is that the complex function controlled or executed by the system is not localized in any one of its parts. The function is a property of the dynamic activity within the system: it resides in the system as such. Part functions, or simple aspects of system function, may be executed by local operations in restricted parts of such a system. This may explain why local lesions of a distributed system scarcely ever destroy system function completely, but degrade it to an extent determined by lesion size and the critical role of the locus destroyed for system function. The remarkable capacity for improvement of function after partial brain lesions is viewed as evidence for the adaptive capacity of such distributed systems to achieve a behavioral goal, albeit slowly and with error, with the remaining neural apparatus.

Finally, distributed systems are by definition and observation both reentrant systems and linkages to inflow and outflow channels of the nervous system. This suggests that the large numbers of processing modules in the neocortex are accessible to both internally generated and externally induced neural activity. Phasic cycling of internally generated activity, accessing first primary sensory but then successively more general and abstract processing units of the homotypical cortex, should allow a continual updating of the perceptual image of self and self-in-the-world as well as a matching function between that perceptual image and impinging external events. This internal readout of internally stored information, and its match with the neural replication of the external continuum, is thought to provide an objective mechanism for conscious awareness. That mechanism is not beyond the reach of scientific enquiry.

References

Abeles, M., and M.H. Goldstein, 1970. Functional architecture in cat primary auditory cortex: Columnar organization and organization according to depth. *J. Neurophysiol.* 33:172-187.

Anderssen, P., P.J. Hagan, C.G. Phillips, and T.P.S. Powell, 1975. Mapping by microstimulation of overlapping projections from area 4 to motor units of the baboon's hand. *Proc. R. Soc. Lond.* B188:31-88.

Armstrong-James, M., 1975. The functional status and columnar organization of single cells responding to cutaneous stimulation in neonatal rat somatosensory cortex S-I. *J. Physiol.* 246:501-538.

Asanuma, H., 1973. Cerebral cortical control of movement. *Physiologist* 16:143-166.

Asanuma, H., 1975. Recent developments in the study of the columnar arrangement of neurons in the motor cortex. *Physiol. Rev.* 55:143-156.

Asanuma, H., and I. Rosen, 1972a. Functional role of afferent input to the monkey motor cortex. *Brain Res.* 40:3-5.

Asanuma, H., and I. Rosen, 1972b. Topographical organization of cortical efferent zones projecting to distal forelimb muscles in the monkey. *Exp. Brain Res.* 14:243-256.

Asanuma, H., and I. Rosen, 1973. Spread of mono- and polysynaptic connections within cat's motor cortex. *Exp. Brain Res.* 16:507-520.

Barlow, H.B., C. Blakemore, and J.D. Pettigrew, 1967. The neural mechanisms of binocular depth discrimination. *J. Physiol.* 193:327-342.

Berrevoets, C.E., and H.G.J.M. Kuypers, 1975. Pericruciate cortical neurons projecting to brain stem reticular formation, dorsal column nuclei, and spinal cord in cat. *Neurosci. Letters* 1: 257-262.

Bok, S.T., 1959. *Histonomy of the Cerebral Cortex*. Princeton: Van Nostrand-Reinhold.

Bonin, B. von, and P. Bailey, 1947. *The Neocortex of Macaca Mulatta*. Urbana: University of Illinois Press.

Brugge, J.F., and M.M. Merzenich, 1973. Responses of neurons in auditory cortex of the macaque monkey to monaural and binaural stimulation. *J. Neurophysiol.* 36:1138–1158.

Carli, G., R.H. LaMotte, and V.B. Mountcastle, 1971a. A comparison of sensory behavior and the activity of postcentral cortical neurons, observed simultaneously, elicited by oscillating mechanical stimuli delivered to the contralateral hand in monkeys. *Proc. 25th Int. Cong. Physiol.*

Carli, G., R.H. LaMotte, and V.B. Mountcastle, 1971b. A simultaneous study of somatic sensory behavior and the activity of somatic sensory cortical neurons. *Fed. Proc.* 30:664.

Carreras, M., and S.A. Andersson, 1963. Functional properties of neurons of the anterior ectosylvian gyrus of the cat. *J. Neurophysiol.* 26:100–126.

Celesia, G.G., 1976. Organization of auditory cortical areas in man. *Brain* 99:403–414.

Colonnier, M., 1966. The structural design of the neocortex. In *Brain and Conscious Experience*, J.C. Eccles, ed. New York: Springer-Verlag, pp. 1–23.

Colonnier, M., 1968. Synaptic patterns on different cell types and the different laminae of the cat visual cortex. An electron-microscope study. *Brain Res.* 9:268–287.

Creutzfeldt, O., 1976. The brain as a functional entity. *Prog. Brain Res.* 45:451–462.

Doetsch, G.S., and E.B. Gardner, 1972. Relationship between afferent input and motor output in sensorimotor cortex of the monkey. *Exp. Neurol.* 35:78–97.

Dryer, D.A., P.R. Loe, C.B. Metz, and B.L. Whitsel, 1975. Representation of head and face in postcentral gyrus of the macaque. *J. Neurophysiol.* 38:714–733.

Duffy, F.H., and J.L. Burchfiel, 1971. Somatosensory system: Organizational hierarchy from single units in monkey area 5. *Science* 172:273–275.

Evarts, E.V., 1964. Temporal patterns of discharge of pyramidal tract neurons during sleep and waking in the monkey. *J. Neurophysiol.* 27:152–171.

Evarts, E.V., 1974. Precentral and postcentral cortical activity in association with visually triggered movements. *J. Neurophysiol.* 37:373–381.

Evarts, E.V., 1975. The Third Stevenson Lecture. Changing concepts of central control of movement. *Can. J. Physiol. Pharmacol.* 53:191–201.

Feldman, M.L., and A. Peters, 1974. A study of barrels and pyramidal dendritic clusters in the cerebral cortex. *Brain Res.* 77:55–76.

Fisken, R.A., L.J. Garey, and T.P.S. Powell, 1973. Patterns of degeneration after intrinsic lesions of the visual cortex (area 17) of the monkey. *Brain Res.* 51:208–213.

Garey, L.J., 1976. Synaptic organization of afferent fibres and intrinsic circuits in the neo-cortex. In *Handbook of EEG Clin. Neurophysiol.*, Vol. 2, Pt. A, Sect. IV, A. Remond, ed. Amsterdam: Elsevier, pp. 57–85.

Garey, L.J., and T.P.S. Powell, 1971. An experimental study of the termination of the lateral geniculo-cortical pathways in the cat and the monkey. *Proc. R. Soc. Lond.* B179:41–63.

Gatter, K.C., D.A. Winfield, and T.P.S. Powell, 1977. The neurons of the cortex of areas 4 and 17 in the cat and rat. In preparation.

Gilbert, C.D., and J.P. Kelly, 1975. The projections of cells in different layers of the cat's visual cortex. *J. Comp. Neurol.* 163:81–106.

Glickstein, M., and D. Whitteridge, 1976. Degeneration of layer III pyramidal cells in area 18 following destruction of callosal input. *Brain Res.* 104:148–151.

Goldman, P., and W.J.H. Nauta, 1976a. Autoradiographic demonstration of cortico-cortical columns in the motor, frontal association, and limbic cortex of the developing rhesus monkey. *Neurosci. Abstr.*, p. 136.

Goldman, P., and W.J.H. Nauta, 1976b. An intricately patterned prefrontocaudate projection in the rhesus monkey. *J. Comp. Neurol.* 171:369–385.

Goldman, P.S., and W.J.H. Nauta, 1977. Columnar distribution of cortico-cortical fibers in the frontal association, limbic, and motor cortex of the developing rhesus monkey. *Brain Res.* 122:393–413.

Grant, G., S. Landgren, and H. Silvenius, 1975. Columnar distribution of U-fibres from the postcruciate cerebral projection area of the cat's group I muscle afferents. *Exp. Brain Res.* 24:57–74.

Hodos, W., 1970. Evolutionary interpretation of neural and behavioral studies of living verte-brates. In *The Neurosciences: Second Study Program*, F.O. Schmitt, ed. New York: Rocke-feller University Press.

Hubel, D.H., and T.N. Wiesel, 1968. Receptive fields and functional architecture of monkey striate cortex. *J. Physiol.* 195:215–243.

Hubel, D.H., and T.N. Wiesel, 1970. Cells sensitive to binocular depth in area 18 of the macaque monkey cortex. *Nature* (Lond.) 225:41–72.

Hubel, D.H., and T.N. Wiesel, 1972. Laminar and columnar distribution of geniculo-cortical fibers in the macaque monkey. *J. Comp. Neurol.* 146:421–450.

Hubel, D.H., and T.N. Wiesel, 1974a. Sequence, regularity and geometry of orientation columns in the monkey striate cortex. *J. Comp. Neurol.* 158:267–294.

Hubel, D.H., and T.N. Wiesel, 1974b. Uniformity of monkey striate cortex: A parallel relation-ship between field size, scatter, and magnification factor. *J. Comp. Neurol.* 158:295–305.

Hubel, D.H., and T.N. Wiesel, 1977. Functional architecture of macaque monkey cortex. *Proc. R. Soc. Lond.* B198:1–59.

Humphrey, D.R., and R.R. Rietz, 1976. Cells of origin of corticorubral projections from the arm area of primate motor cortex and their synaptic actions in the red nucleus. *Brain Res.* 110:162–169.

Hyvärinen, J., and A. Poranen, 1974. Function of the parietal associative area 7 as revealed from cellular discharges in alert monkeys. *Brain* 97:673–692.

Imig, T.J., and H.O. Adrian, 1977. Binaural columns in the primary (AI) of cat auditory cortex. *Brain Res.* (in press).

Jacobsen, S., and J.Q. Trojanowski, 1977. Prefrontal granular cortex of the rhesus monkey. II. Interhemispheric cortical afferents. *Brain Res.* 132:235–246.

Jankowska, E., Y. Padel, and R. Tanaka, 1975a. The mode of activation of pyramidal tract cells by intracortical stimuli. *J. Physiol.* 249:617–636.

Jankowska, E., Y. Padel, and R. Tanaka, 1975b. Projections of pyramidal tract cells to alpha-motoneurons innervating hand-limb muscles in monkey. *J. Physiol.* 249:636–667.

Jerison, H.J., 1973. *Evolution of the Brain and Intelligence.* New York: Academic Press.

Jones, E.G., 1975a. Lamination and differential distribution of thalamic afferents within the sensory motor cortex of the squirrel monkey. *J. Comp. Neurol.* 160:167–204.

Jones, E.G., 1975b. Varieties and distribution of non-pyramidal cells in the somatic sensory cortex of the squirrel monkey. *J. Comp. Neurol.* 160:205–267.

Jones, E.G., and H. Burton, 1976. Areal differences in the laminar distribution of thalamic afferents in cortical fields of the insular, parietal and temporal regions of primates. *J. Comp. Neurol.* 168:197–247.

Jones, E.G., H. Burton, and R. Porter, 1975. Commissural and cortico-cortical "columns" in the somatic sensory cortex of primates. *Science* 190:572–574.

Jones, E.G., J.D. Coulter, H. Burton, and R. Porter, 1977. Cells of origin and terminal distribution of corticostriatal fibers arising in the sensory motor cortex of monkeys. *J. Comp. Neurol.* 173:53–80.

Jones, E.G., and T.P.S. Powell, 1970. An electron microscopic study of the laminar pattern and mode of termination of afferent fibre pathways in the somatic sensory cortex of the cat. *Phil. Trans. R. Soc. Lond.* B257:1–11.

Jones, E.G., and S.P. Wise, 1977. Size, laminar and columnar distribution of efferent cells in the sensory-motor cortex of primates. *J. Comp. Neurol.* 175:391–438.

Knight, P.L., 1977. Representation of the cochlea within the anterior auditory field (AAF) of the cat. *Brain Res.* 130:447–467.

Kunzle, H., 1976. Alternating afferent zones of high and low axon terminal density within the macaque motor cortex. *Brain Res.* 106:365–370.

Lashley, K.S., 1949. Persistent problems in the evolution of mind. *Quart. Rev. Biol.* 24:28–42.

Lashley, K.S., and G. Clark, 1946. The cytoarchitecture of the cerebral cortex of Ateles: A critical examination of cytoarchitectonic studies. *J. Comp. Neurol.* 85:223–305.

Lenon, R.N., and R. Porter, 1976. Afferent input to movement-related precentral neurones in conscious monkeys. *Proc. R. Soc. Lond.* B194:313–339.

LeVay, S., 1973. Synaptic patterns in the visual cortex of the cat and monkey. Electron microscopy of Golgi preparations. *J. Comp. Neurol.* 150:53–86.

Lorente de Nó, R., 1938. Cerebral cortex: Architecture, intracortical connections, motor projections. In *Physiology of the Nervous System*, J.F. Fulton, ed. New York: Oxford University Press, pp. 291–339.

Lund, J.S., 1973. Organization of neurons in the visual cortex area 17 of the monkey *(Macaca mulatta)*. *J. Comp. Neurol.* 147:455–496.

Lund, J.S. and R.G. Boothe, 1975. Interlaminar connections and pyramidal neuron organization in the visual cortex, area 17, of the macaque monkey. *J. Comp. Neurol.* 159:305–334.

Lund, J.S., R.D. Lund, A.E. Hendrickson, A.H. Bunt, and A.F. Fuchs, 1975. The origin of efferent pathways from the primary visual cortex, area 17, of the macaque monkey as shown by retrograde transport of horseradish peroxidase. *J. Comp. Neurol.* 164:287–304.

Lynch, J.C., C. Acuna, H. Sakata, A. Georgopoulos, and V.B. Mountcastle, 1973a. The parietal association area and immediate extrapersonal space. *Proc. Soc. Neurosci.*

Lynch, J.C., H. Sakata, A. Georgopoulos, and V.B. Mountcastle, 1973b. Parietal association cortex neurons active during hand and eye tracking of objects in immediate extrapersonal space. *Physiologist* 16:384.

Lynch, J.C., V.B. Mountcastle, W.H. Talbot, and T.C.T. Yin, 1977. Parietal lobe mechanisms of directed visual attention. *J. Neurophysiol.* 40:362–389.

Marin-Padilla, M., 1969. Origin of the pericellular baskets of the pyramidal cells of the human motor cortex: A Golgi study. *Brain Res.* 14:633–646.

Marin-Padilla, M., 1970. Prenatal and early postnatal ontogenesis of the human motor cortex: A Golgi study. II. The basket-pyramidal system. *Brain Res.* 23:185–191.

Meller, K., and W. Tetzlaff, 1975. Neuronal migration during the early development of the cerebral cortex: A scanning electron microscopic study. *Cell Tissue Res.* 163:313–325.

Merzenich, M.M., and J.F. Brugge, 1973. Representation of the cochlear partition on the superior temporal plane of the macaque monkey. *Brain Res.* 50:275–296.

Merzenich, M.M., P.L. Knight, and G.L. Roth, 1975. Representation of cochlea within primary auditory cortex in the cat. *J. Neurophysiol.* 38:231–249.

Molliver, M.E., R. Grzanna, J.H. Morison, and J.T. Coyle, 1977. Immunohistochemical characterization of noradrenergic innervation in the rat neocortex: A regional and laminar analysis. *Neurosci. Abstr.*

Moore, R.Y., and F.E. Bloom, 1977. Central catecholamine neuron systems: Anatomy and physiology. *Annu. Rev. Neurosci.* (in press).

Mountcastle, V.B., 1957. Modality and topographic properties of single neurons of cat's somatic sensory cortex. *J. Neurophysiol.* 20:408–434.

Mountcastle, V.B., 1975. The view from within: Pathways to the study of perception. *Johns Hopkins Med. J.* 136:109–131.

Mountcastle, V.B., 1976. The world around us: Neural command functions for selective attention. The F.O. Schmitt Lecture for 1975. *Neurosci. Res. Program Bull.* 14 (Suppl. 1).

Mountcastle, V.B., 1977. Brain mechanisms for directed attention. The Sherrington Memorial Lecture. *Proc. R. Soc. Med.* (in press).

Mountcastle, V.B., J.C. Lynch, A. Georgopoulos, H. Sakata, and A. Acuna, 1975. Posterior parietal association cortex of the monkey: Command functions for operations within extrapersonal space. *J. Neurophysiol.* 38:871–908.

Mountcastle, V.B., and T.P.S. Powell, 1959a. Central nervous mechanisms subserving position sense and kinesthesis. *Bull. Johns Hopkins Hosp.* 105:173–200.

Mountcastle, V.B., and T.P.S. Powell, 1959b. Neural mechanisms subserving cutaneous sensibility, with special reference to the role of afferent inhibition in sensory perception and discrimination. *Bull. Johns Hopkins Hosp.* 105:201–232.

Mountcastle, V.B., W.H. Talbot, H. Sakata, and J. Hyvärinen, 1969. Cortical neuronal mechanisms studied in unanesthetized monkeys. Neuronal periodicity and frequency discrimination. *J. Neurophysiol.* 32:454–484.

Nikara, T., P.O. Ship, and J.C. Pettigrew, 1968. Analysis of retinal correspondence by studying receptive fields of binocular single units in cat striate cortex. *Exp. Brain Res.* 6:353–372.

Parker, D.E., 1965. Vertical organization in the auditory cortex of the cat. *J. Audit. Res.* 2: 99–124.

Pasternak, J.R., and T.A. Woolsey, 1975. The number, size, and spatial distribution of neurons in lamina IV of the mouse SMI neocortex. *J. Comp. Neurol.* 160:291–306.

Paul, R.L., M. Merzenich, and H. Goodman, 1972. Representation of slowly and rapidly adapting cutaneous mechanoreceptors of the hand in Brodmann's areas 3 and 1 of *Macaca mulatta*. *Brain Res.* 36:229–249.

Pettigrew, J.D., T. Nikara, and P.O. Bishop, 1968. Binocular interaction on single units in cat striate cortex: Simultaneous stimulation by single moving slit with receptive fields in correspondence. *Exp. Brain Res.* 6:391–410.

Phillips. C.C., 1969. Motor apparatus of the baboon's hand. *Proc. R. Soc. Lond.* B173:141–174.

Poggio, G.F., F.H. Baker, R.J.W. Mansfield, A. Sillito, and P. Grigg, 1975. Spatial and chromatic properties of neurons subserving foveal and parafoveal vision in rhesus monkey. *Brain Res.* 100:25–59.

Poggio, G.F., R.W. Doty, Jr., and W.H. Talbot, 1977. Foveal striate cortex of the behaving monkey. Single neuron responses to square-wave gratings during fixation of gaze. *J. Neurophysiol.* 40:1369-1391.

Poggio, G.F., and B. Fisher, 1977. Binocular interaction and depth sensitivity of striate and prestriate cortical neurons of the behaving rhesus monkey. *J. Neurophysiol.* 40:1392-1405.

Powell, T.P.S., and V.B. Mountcastle, 1959. Some aspects of the functional organization of the cortex of the postcentral gyrus of the monkey: A correlation of findings obtained in a single unit analysis with cytoarchitecture. *Bull. Johns Hopkins Hosp.* 105:133-162.

Powell, T.P.S., and V.B. Mountcastle, 1977. Unpublished observations of a series of fetal monkey brains kindly supplied by D. Bodian.

Radinsky, L.B., 1967. Relative brain size: A new measure. *Science* 155:836-837.

Raichle, M.E., B.K. Hartman, J.O. Eichling, and L.G. Sharpe, 1975. Central adrenergic regulation of cerebral blood flow and vascular permeability. *Proc. Natl. Acad. Sci. USA* 72:3726-3730.

Rakic, P., 1971. Guidance of neurons migrating to the fetal monkey neocortex. *Brain Res.* 33:471-476.

Rakic, P., 1972. Mode of cell migration to the superficial layers of fetal monkey neocortex. *J. Comp. Neurol.* 145:61-84.

Rakic, P., 1974. Neurons in rhesus monkey visual cortex: Systematic relation between time of origin and eventual disposition. *Science* 183:425-427.

Rakic, P., 1975. Timing of major ontogenetic events in the visual cortex of the rhesus monkey. In *Brain Mechanisms in Mental Retardation*, J. Buchwald and M. Brazier, eds. New York: Academic Press.

Rakic, P., 1977. Prenatal development of the visual system in rhesus monkey. *Philos. Trans. R. Soc. Lond.* B278:245-260.

Rakic, P., 1978. Neuronal migration and contact guidance in the primate telencephalon. *Postgrad. Med. J.* (in press).

Rockel, A.J., R.W. Hiorns, and T.P.S. Powell, 1974. Numbers of neurons through full depth of neocortex. *Proc. Anat. Soc. Gr. Br. Ire.* 118:371.

Rose, J.E., 1949. The cellular structure of the auditory region of the cat. *J. Comp. Neurol.* 91:409-440.

Rose, J.E., and C.N. Woolsey, 1948a. Structure and relations of limbic cortex and anterior thalamic nuclei in rabbit and cat. *J. Comp. Neurol.* 89:279-348.

Rose, J.E., and C.N. Woolsey, 1948b. The orbitofrontal cortex and its connections with the mediodorsal nucleus in rabbit, sheep and cat. *Assoc. Res. Nerv. Ment. Dis.* 27:210-232.

Rose, J.E., and C.N. Woolsey, 1949. The relations of thalamic connections, cellular structure and evocable electrical activity in the auditory region of the cat. *J. Comp. Neurol.* 91:441-466.

Sacher, G.A., 1970. Allometric and factorial analysis of brain structure in insectivores and primates. In *The Primate Brain*, C.R. Noback and W. Montagna, eds. New York: Appleton-Century-Crofts, pp. 245–287.

Sakata, H., Y. Takaoka, A. Kawarasaki, and H. Shibutani, 1973. Somatosensory properties of neurons in the superior parietal cortex (area 5) of the rhesus monkey. *Brain Res.* 64:85–102.

Schmechel, D.E., and P. Rakic, 1973. Evolution of fetal radial glial cells in rhesus monkey telencephalon. A Golgi study. *Anat. Rec.* 175:436.

Schmitt, F.O., P. Dev., and B.H. Smith, 1976. Electrotonic processing of information by brain cells. *Science* 193:114–120.

Shanks, M.F., R.C.A. Pearson, and T.P.S. Powell, 1977. The intrinsic connections of the primary sensory cortex of the monkey. *Proc. R. Soc. Lond.* (in press).

Shanks, M.F., A.J. Rockel, and T.P.S. Powell, 1975. The commissural fibre connections of the primary somatic sensory cortex. *Brain Res.* 98:166–171.

Shoumura, K., 1974. An attempt to relate the origin and distribution of commisural fibres to the presence of large and medium pyramids in layer III in the cat's visual cortex. *Brain Res.* 67:13–25.

Shoumura, K., T. Ando, and K. Kato, 1975. Structural organization of "callosal" OBg in human corpus callosum agenesis. *Brain Res.* 93:241–252.

Sidman, R.L., 1970. Autoradiographic methods and principles for study of the nervous system with thymidine-H^3. In *Contemporary Research Techniques in Neuroanatomy*, O.E. Ebbesson and W.J.H. Nauta, eds. New York: Springer-Verlag.

Sidman, R.L., and P. Rakic, 1973. Neuronal migration, with special reference to developing human brain: A review. *Brain Res.* 62:1–35.

Sloper, J.J., 1973. An electron microscope study of the termination of afferent connections to the primate motor cortex. *J. Neurocytol.* 2:361–368.

Sousa-Pinta, A., 1973. The structure of the first auditory cortex (AI) in the cat. I. Light microscopic observations on its organization. *Arch. Ital. Biol.* 111:112–137.

Stephan, H., 1967. Quantitative Vergleiche zur phylogenetischen Entwicklung des Gehirns der Primaten mit Hilfe von Progressionindices. *Mitt. Max-Planck-Ges.* 2:63–86.

Stephen, H., 1969. Quantitative investigations on visual structures in primate brains. In *Proc. 2nd Int. Cong. Primat.* Vol. 3: *Neurology, Physiology, and Infectious Diseases*, H.O. Hofer, ed. Basel: Karger, pp. 34–42.

Stephan, H., 1972. Evolution of primate brains: A comparative anatomical investigation. In *The Functional and Evolutionary Biology of Primates*, T. Tuttle, ed. Chicago: Aldine-Atherton, pp. 155–174.

Stephan, H., and O.J. Andy, 1964. Quantitative comparisons of brain structures from insectivores to primates. *Am. Zool.* 4:59–74.

Stephan, H., and O.J. Andy, 1969. Quantitative comparative neuroanatomy of primates: An attempt at a phylogenetic interpretation. *Ann. NY Acad. Sci.* 167:370–387.

Stephan, H., R. Bauchot, and O.J. Andy, 1970. Data on size of the brain of various brain parts in insectivores and primates. In *The Primate Brain,* C.R. Noback and W. Montagna, eds. New York: Appleton-Century-Crofts, pp. 289–297.

Stephanis, C., and H. Jasper, 1964. Recurrent collateral inhibition in pyramidal tract neurons. *J. Neurophysiol.* 27:855–877.

Suga, N., 1977. Amplitude spectrum representation in the Doppler-shifted CF processing area of the auditory cortex of the mustache bat. *Science* 196:64–67.

Szentágothai, J., 1973. Synaptology of the visual cortex. In *Visual Centers of the Brain (Handbook of Sensory Physiology,* Vol. VII/3), R. Jung, ed. Berlin-New York:Springer-Verlag.

Szentágothai, J., 1975. The 'module-concept' in cerebral cortex architecture. *Brain Res.* 95: 475–496.

Szentágothai, J., 1976. Basic circuitry of the neocortex. *Exp. Brain Res.* (Suppl. 1):282–287.

Szentágothai, J., and M.A. Arbib, 1974. Conceptual models of neural organization. *Neurosci. Res. Program Bull.* 12:307–510.

Tömböl, T., 1974. An electron microscopic study of the neurons of the visual cortex. *J. Neurocytol.* 3:525–531.

Towe, A.L., 1975. Notes on the hypothesis of columnar organization in somatosensory cortex. *Brain Behav. Evol.* 11:16–47.

Tunturi, A.R., 1952. A difference in the representation of auditory signals for the left and right ears in the iso-frequency contours of the right middle ectosylvian auditory cortex of the dog. *Am. J. Physiol.* 168:712–727.

Tunturi, A.R., and J.A. Dudman, 1958. Model of storage space in the MES auditory cortex. *Am. J. Physiol.* 192:437–446.

Washburn, S.L., and R.S. Harding, 1970. Evolution of primate behavior. In *The Neurosciences: Second Study Program,* F.O. Schmitt, ed. New York: Rockefeller University Press, pp. 39–47.

Welker, C., 1971. Microelectrode delineation of fine grain somatotopic organization of SMI cerebral neocortex in albino rat. *Brain Res.* 26:259–275.

Werner, G., and B.L. Whitsel, 1968. Topology of the body representation in somatosensory I of primates. *J. Neurophysiol.* 31:856–869.

Werner, G., and B.L. Whitsel, 1973. The somatic sensory cortex: Functional organization. In *The Somatosensory System (Handbook of Sensory Physiology,* Vol. II), A. Iggo, ed. Berlin-New York:Springer-Verlag.

Whitsel, B.L., and D.A. Dreyer, 1976. Comparison of single unit data obtained from the different topographic subdivisions of the postcentral gyrus of the macaque: Implications for the organization of somatosensory projection pathways. *Exp. Brain Res.* (Suppl. 1):415–420.

Whitsel, B.L., D.A. Dreyer, and J.R. Ropollo, 1971. Determinants of the body representation in the postcentral gyrus of macaques. *J. Neurophysiol.* 34:1018.

Whitsel, B.L., L.M. Petrucelli, and G. Werner, 1969. Symmetry and connectivity in the map of the body surface in somatosensory area II of primates. *J. Neurophysiol.* 32:170–183.

Whitsel, B.L., J.R. Ropollo, and G. Werner, 1972. Cortical information processing of stimulus motion on primate skin. *J. Neurophysiol.* 35:691–717.

Winfield, D.A., and T.P.S. Powell, 1976. The termination of thalamo-cortical fibres in the visual cortex of the cat. *J. Neurocytol.* 5:269–281.

Woolsey, C.N., 1960. Organization of cortical auditory system. In *Neural Mechanisms of the Auditory and Vestibular Systems*, G.L. Rasmussen and W.F. Windle, eds. Springfield, Ill.: Thomas.

Woolsey, T.A., and H. Van Der Loos, 1970. The structural organization of layer IV in the somatosensory region (SI) of mouse cerebral cortex. The description of a cortical field composed of discrete cytoarchitectural units. *Brain Res.* 17:205–242.

Woolsey, T.A., C. Welker, and R.H. Schwartz, 1975. Comparative anatomical studies of the SMI face cortex with special reference to the occurrence of 'barrels' in layer IV. *J. Comp. Neurol.* 164:79–94.

Zeki, S., 1974. The mosaic organization of the visual cortex in the monkey. In *A Festschrift for Professor J.Z. Young*, R. Bellairs and E.G. Gray, eds. London: Oxford University Press, pp. 327–343.

Zeki, S.M., 1975. The functional organization of projections from striate to prestriate visual cortex in the rhesus monkey. *Cold Spring Harbor Symp. Quant. Biol.* 40:591–600.

Zeki, S.M., 1977. Colour coding in the superior temporal sulcus of rhesus monkey visual cortex. *Proc. R. Soc. Lond.* (in press).

GROUP SELECTION AND PHASIC REENTRANT SIGNALING: A THEORY OF HIGHER BRAIN FUNCTION

Gerald M. Edelman

Introduction

The remarkable diversity of nervous systems in various animal species and their exquisite capacity for adaptive function are both intriguing and confounding to neurobiologists. Despite their complexity, however, all nervous systems appear to obey similar general principles at the level of morphological expression of neuronal structures and in their mechanisms of signal transmission. The recognition of these general principles and their application to the study of simple nervous systems as well as to subsystems in more complex brains have been among the greatest triumphs of neurobiology in this century (Quarton, Melnechuk, and Schmitt, 1967; Schmitt, 1970; Schmitt and Worden, 1974; Kuffler and Nicholls, 1977).

At the functional level, however, fundamental and methodological confusion still reigns. In many cases, the function of subsystems is only obscurely defined. Indeed, for higher brain functions expressed in perception, in awareness or consciousness, and in complex cognitive acts, the relation of nervous system structure and function has until recently (Eccles, 1966a) been a ground left mainly to philosophical speculation. At best, it has been the subject of psychological investigation under a variety of deliberately limited paradigms such as classical or instrumental conditioning, genetic epistemology, or linguistic analysis (Herrnstein and Bornig, 1965; Skinner, 1966; Piaget, 1950, 1954; Lenneberg, 1970). These efforts, while worthy, do not directly address the most challenging problem of neurobiology: the determination of the structural substrates and cellular mechanisms of higher brain functions, particularly those underlying consciousness.

Recent progress in the analysis of perception prompts the hope that the situation will improve in the next several decades. The pioneering studies of Mountcastle (1957, 1967) on sensory processing, of Hubel and Wiesel (1974) on visual processing, and of Sperry (1970a) on localization of brain function in the cerebral hemispheres are major developments relating cellular and neuronal activities to the performance of complex perceptual and conceptual tasks.

Despite these developments, the higher-order neural processing that leads to thinking, consciousness, and preparation for future acts has not been satisfactorily described in terms that explicitly take into account the details of brain structure. This is hardly surprising; the complexity of mammalian neuronal systems and their behavioral repertoires is enormous, and it would be premature to elaborate a detailed theory to account for their function. It may not be premature, however, to ask a more general question related to the evolution, development, and function of higher brain systems, particularly those in man: Does the brain operate according to a single principle in carrying out its higher-order cognitive functions? That is, despite the manifold differences in brain subsystems and the particularities of their connections, can one discern a general mechanism or principle that is required for the realization of cognitive faculties? If so, at what level does the mechanism operate—cells, molecules, or circuits of cells?

It is my purpose here to suggest such a principle on both theoretical and experimental grounds. After describing this principle and relating it to some of the available facts, I shall consider its application to an understanding of higher brain states with an emphasis on consciousness. The basic idea is that the brain is a *selective* system that processes sensorimotor information through the temporally coordinated interactions of collections or repertoires of functionally equivalent units each consisting of a small group of neurons. According to the model developed here, the brain processes sensory signals and its own stored information upon this selective base in a phasic (cyclic) and reentrant manner that is capable of generating the necessary conditions for conscious states.

In constructing a theory to account for higher brain function, several minimal criteria must be met:

1. The theory must be consistent with neuroanatomical, embryological, and neurophysiological information.

2. It must account for the distributive properties of memory and learning, for associative recall, as well as for the temporal properties and temporal "scale" of recall.

3. It must permit updating of memory to accord with current inputs.

4. It must reflect the main functions of higher brain systems as mediators between action and experience.

5. It must provide the necessary, if not the sufficient, conditions for awareness.

A number of theories meet some of these criteria but not all. Moreover, no current theory attempts to relate the embryonic development of the brain to its mature higher functions in any consistent fashion. This will be one of the major goals of the present formulation. At the same time, the theory will be couched in terms that are as general as possible. While this will result in a neuroanatomically impoverished model, in the sense that most circuit details will be left out, a deliberate effort will be made to avoid abstract model building that generates functional properties without reference to the nervous system.

Selection and Its Premises

In order to understand the idea of selection, it is useful to consider two extreme modes of possible brain function. In the first mode, the higher brain centers are connected in a rigorously defined and determinate fashion (Brodal, 1975), but they cannot function until properly transduced and processed sensory inputs instruct the circuitry to undergo stable changes in an equally unambiguous and determinate fashion. This instruction could operate at the level of molecules, synapses, cells (particularly cell membranes), or large groups of cells. The instructional mode has two characteristics: (1) the informational structure of the outside signal is primary and therefore necessary for the elaboration of the appropriately coded brain structure and for its function; and (2) there are no prior or preexisting states of the brain structure already capable of processing such a signal. Instruction implies that the interaction between brain structures and the first presentation of the signal is unique and determinate; that is, only following the signal input is a functioning brain structure or circuit formed that uniquely "corresponds" to sensory information of that kind.

Such an instructive model of higher brain function faces a number of difficulties. Instruction requires a precise mapping of corresponding information at either the molecular level (in terms of templates, for example) or the cellular level (in terms of an unambiguous and stable code). For instruction to occur, it would be necessary for each complex sensory event to result in storage of a particular *precise* complementary pattern that did not previously exist in the molecules or cells of the brain. New sensory events with some elements in common with previous events would have to share components of previous patterns or else lay down entirely new corresponding patterns. In the former case, successive experiences would require a higher-order mechanism for distinguishing old elements from new, and in the latter, the risk of exhausting the informational potential of the system would be great.

In general, the information that is processed in the brain arrives as a set of electrical or chemical signals whose molecular modes of production are already specified. It is difficult to understand on chemical grounds how either action potentials, graded potentials, or chemical transmitters could directly specify a stable pattern of complex coded information in macromolecules. Moreover, groups of cells cannot easily be "templated"—a variety of genetic, epigenetic, and transient alterations that are known to occur would threaten the stability of any unique circuit set up by outside instruction. Finally, an instructive theory of brain function would give no basis for understanding apparently autonomous higher activities such as conscious awareness and the creative programming of future events. In a sense, it puts the brain too much at the mercy of the outside world.

The alternative view is that the brain is a selective system, a proposal made by several authors, but without extensive elaboration (Jerne, 1967; Edelman, 1975; Young, 1975). Although the meaning of "selective" is best made clear by considering the detailed requirements of such a system, it may be useful to start off with a preliminary definition. "Selection" implies that after ontogeny and early development, the brain contains cellular configurations that can already respond discriminatingly to outside signals because of their genetically determined structures or because of epigenetic alterations that have occurred independently of the structure of outside signals. These signals serve merely to select among preexisting configurations of cells or cell groups in order to create an appropriate response.

Such selective notions have been prevalent in different forms in both evolutionary theory and immunology (Edelman, 1974a) and are understood in greater or lesser detail. The project I have set myself here, however, is not simply to make comparisons or analogies among these systems, but rather to explore whether a particular form of selection provides a basis for explaining higher brain function. A consideration of the general requirements and consequences of the operation of selective systems is nonetheless important, and in this context, occasional comparisons with other systems may be useful.

Before discussing these requirements, it is necessary to specify briefly the level at which selection acts as well as to justify the theoretical need for selective mechanisms of brain function. Accordingly, the proposals made here rest on one experimental premise and one theoretical premise:

1. The main unit of function and selection in the higher brain is a group of cells (consisting of perhaps 50–10,000 neurons) connected in a large variety of ways but not necessarily in accord with the assumptions of the classical neuron doctrine (Bullock, 1959; Bodian, 1962). The grounds for altering these assumptions have been reviewed by Shepherd (1972) on the basis of work on the olfactory bulb and the retina. Additional evidence to support the cell group as the unit of selection comes from the work of Mountcastle (1957, 1967) and Hubel and Wiesel (1974), demonstrating both the existence and function of columns or slabs of cortical cells in sensory projection areas. A further (and so far hypothetical) assumption made here is that, in certain cortical areas, these groups of cells need not be connected in an absolutely fixed fashion from animal to animal and region to region; instead, local circuit neurons (LCNs) provide a very large variety of ways in which groups of cells may be connected both electrically and chemically (Schmitt, Dev, and Smith, 1976). A useful distinction may be made here. *Intrinsic connections* exist within a neuronal group and may involve a variety of modes of interaction within a local circuit, including all modes of nonsynaptic interaction. *Extrinsic connections* include all those outside a neuronal group, particularly those between groups. It is mainly at the level of intrinsic connections that we assume great variability from group to group. Although some variability of extrinsic connections may exist, it is clear that at this level, the connectivity of the brain is quite specific and highly architectonic.

2. The nervous system of animals capable of carrying out complex sensorimotor acts can successfully adapt to complexes of informational input that have never before been encountered in the history of an individual or of its species. This premise is difficult to prove but is probably most defensible in man. Perhaps the most dramatic examples are the capabilities of some individuals to solve highly abstract problems in mathematics, to generate new symbol structures of the complexity of a symphony, or to analyze such unique structures in a surprisingly efficient fashion upon seeing them for the first time.

This extraordinary capacity poses problems for both instructive and selective theories. On the surface, instructive theories can evade the problem by posing successive templates at higher and higher levels in the hierarchical organization of the brain; but this merely makes such theories seem all the more unlikely. On the other hand, to account for such grand feats of information processing, selective theories might be required to posit a very large repertoire of different preexisting functional units or neuronal groups. Is such a repertoire possible? In order to answer this question, we must extensively consider the nature and requirements of a selective theory of brain function.

The Requirements of Group Selection and the Need for Degeneracy

It is clear from both evolutionary and immunological theory (Edelman, 1975) that in facing an unknown future, the fundamental requirement for successful adaptation is preexisting diversity. This is achieved in evolution by mutation and gene flow and in immunological systems by a somatically generated antibody repertoire. For the nervous system, we may define a primary repertoire as a diverse collection of neuronal groups whose different functions are already prespecified during ontogeny and development. Without further specification at this point, we shall assume that if a neuronal group responds with characteristic output more or less specifically to an input consisting of a particular spatiotemporal configuration of signals, there is a "match" between that group and the signal configuration. In order to refine further the notion of selection from a repertoire of such neuronal groups, it is essential to consider the general requirements upon such a repertoire, particularly its diversity.

The first requirement is that this repertoire be sufficiently large; that is, it must contain enough diverse elements so that given a wide range of different input signals, a finite probability exists of finding at least one matching element in the repertoire for each signal. Furthermore, for at least some elements of the repertoire, the match with input must be sufficiently specific to distinguish among different input signals (that is, to "recognize" them) with relatively low error. In the case of the immune system, this is accomplished by a repertoire of at least 10^6 different antibody molecules, each with a particular (or sterically defined) antigen-binding site, as well as by certain thresholding mechanisms controlling the immune response (Edelman, 1974b).

What are the general properties of such a large recognition repertoire that would render it capable of both a wide range of recogni-

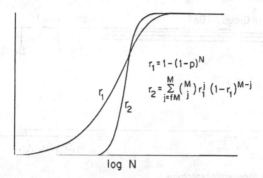

$$r_1 = 1 - (1-p)^N$$

$$r_2 = \sum_{j=fM}^{M} \binom{M}{j} r_1^j (1-r_1)^{M-j}$$

log N

Figure 1. Dependency of two forms of recognition function on the number N of elements in a repertoire, calculated according to a simple model. In this model, each element is assigned a constant a priori probability p of recognizing a randomly chosen signal. Here r_1 represents the expected fraction of all possible signals that will be recognized, and r_2 represents the probability that more than a fraction f (in this case 63%) of the M possible signals will be recognized. The shape of the curve is not sensitive to the value chosen for M if M is large. Similarly, if p is changed, the entire curve shifts left or right, reflecting the altered specificity of recognition, but the shapes of the curves do not change significantly. A more realistic model would assign different p values to different repertoire elements; this would increase the computational complexity, but the nature of the dependency of r upon N would not be fundamentally altered.

tion and specificity for individual signals? First, for any arbitrarily chosen large number of different input signals, there must be a significantly larger number of components in the repertoire (Figure 1). Let a "match" be defined in terms of some threshold of recognition that gives the system the capacity to distinguish two closely related events within certain limits of error. If there are N elements in the repertoire and there is a probability p of a match between any such element and any signal, then we may define a recognition function $r = f(p,N)$ that measures the effectiveness of the system in recognizing a range of possible input signals. Several such functions can be defined, depending upon the particular measure of effectiveness chosen.

Now it is clear that if N is small, then for a large number of different inputs, r will be close to zero. For N above a certain number, r increases until, at some high value of N, a significant increase in the efficacy of matching under the threshold condition can no longer be achieved by a further increase in the size of the repertoire. This suggests that for the central nervous system, N must be large, but in itself it does not help us set any numerical limits. We may assume, however, that in a particular region of the human brain, a repertoire of 10^6 different cell groups, each consisting of 50–10,000 cells, would not exhaust the numbers of cells available.

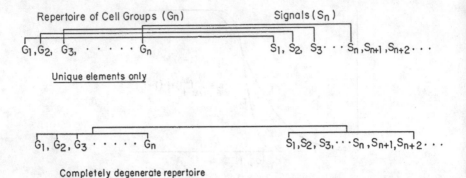

Figure 2. Two extreme cases of repertoires having unique (nondegenerate) and completely degenerate elements. In the first case, extension of the range of signals to be recognized (for example, beyond S_n) leads to a frequent failure of recognition. In the second, there is a loss of specificity and a frequent failure to distinguish different signals inasmuch as each G can respond to all signals.

A key consequence of this analysis is that the selective system for matching a signal or a configuration of signals to the repertoire must be degenerate. By *degeneracy* I mean that, in general, given a particular threshold condition, there must be more than one way of satisfactorily recognizing a given input signal. This implies the presence of multiple neuronal groups with different structures capable of carrying out the same function more or less well. I distinguish degeneracy from *redundancy,* which is used here strictly to imply the presence of repeated units or groups of *identical* structure.

The need for degeneracy is perhaps most easily seen by again assuming extreme cases, one without any degeneracy and the other with complete degeneracy (Figure 2). Consider a repertoire in which, for any one arbitrarily chosen input signal, there is only one cell group capable of recognizing that signal. Under these conditions, in a system capable of recognizing previously unencountered signals, there must ensue a failure of range; that is, many inputs would go unrecognized. If we insist that a wide range of different previously unencountered signals be recognized and distinguished with high frequency by such a repertoire, then the fundamental requirement that there be no participation of the signal in forming the repertoire would have to be breached. Now consider the other extreme—that *every* element in the repertoire match *any* input signal. In this case, the range requirement would be satisfied, but there would be a severe loss of specificity and consequently of the capacity to distinguish between two different but

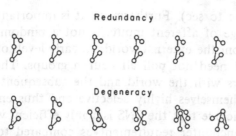

Figure 3. Diagrams illustrating the distinction between redundancy and degeneracy. The structures of degenerate groups carrying out more or less the same function can differ in many respects, sharing only certain common features among their elements: degenerate groups are isofunctional but nonisomorphic. Redundancy is used here in the strict sense: redundant groups are isofunctional and isomorphic.

closely related signal patterns. The composition of the repertoire must therefore be so constituted as to fall between these extremes, so that there are several (and possibly many) different cell groups capable of distinguishing a given input more or less well (that is, sufficiently above the threshold requirement for recognition).

The foregoing analysis suggests that degeneracy is a property fundamental to reconciling specificity of recognition with range of recognition. As we shall see, degeneracy is also consistent with a number of the observed properties of the central nervous systems of man and certain other animal species. As shown in Figure 3, degeneracy is different from strict redundancy but can include redundancy as a special case. Like redundancy, degeneracy can act to provide reliability in a system composed of unreliable components (von Neumann, 1956; Winograd and Cowan, 1963).

Besides these requirements on properties of the repertoire, there is another major requirement for the successful operation of a selective recognition system: a sufficiently large portion of the repertoire must be polled efficiently by various input signals. As in polling a network of computer terminals, the relevant signals must be able to encounter matching elements in the repertoire with a suitably high probability in a sufficiently short time. Moreover, the responses of such elements must be made available to higher-order elements for subsequent recognition events. Obviously this requirement must be met in the CNS by the various connections within and among cell groups. There is no dearth of such connections via either tracts or local circuit neurons, and the efficiency of signal transmission as well as its high signal-to-noise ratio would appear to allow the polling of large numbers of groups in short time periods (msec to sec). Furthermore, it is important to recognize that the total range of afferent inputs is not a random sample of all possible signals from the external world. At early levels of processing, a given input signal need not poll all neuron groups. The interface of sensory transducers with the world and the subsequent processing of their signals are themselves highly selective and thus enhance polling efficiency. We conclude that the CNS is highly efficient with respect to the polling and encounter requirement as compared to the immune system, in which encounter occurs by diffusion, flow, and cell movement.

In addition to the need for a large degenerate repertoire and high encounter probability, there is a third major requirement on a selective system. This is expressed in the need for *amplification* of a selective recognition event so that it can be stored, read out, and reflected stably in a favorable bias of the system for future recognition of the same event. At best, failure of amplification would result in only a transient match after encounter, with a small likelihood that the same selected cell group would be matched in future repetitions of the signal; at worst, it would result in a complete loss of matching in competition with other signals. In the immune system, amplification is achieved by maturation, cell division, and enhanced antibody synthesis by the progeny of selected cells. The net result is a gain of up to 10^5–10^6 in the production of the kind of antibody initially selected and an increase through cell division in the *repertoire frequency* of cells carrying antibodies of that type. In the nervous system, however, there is no neuronal cell division in the mature animal, and amplification presumably must be achieved by synaptic alterations that lead to facilitation of excitation or to suppression of particular pathways. For the present purposes, it is not important whether this occurs by formation of new synaptic contacts or by stable changes at already existing contacts (for example, by membrane changes at dendritic spines or by chemical alterations that change the thresholds of preexisting synaptic connections).

In accord with the amplification requirement, a central assumption in the present theory is that after initial selection, certain cell groups in the repertoire have a higher probability than others of being selected again by a similar or identical signal pattern. This can arise by synaptic facilitation or inhibition of pathways either within a cell group or between cell groups. This change in likelihood either enhances the probability of subsequent selection of some cell groups or reduces the probability that other cell groups will respond. In other words, selection can be either positive or negative. It is important to note, however, that after selection of groups in a degenerate primary repertoire of sufficient size, there would still remain other unselected cell groups of similar specificities. In general, these would have changed probabilities of being encountered and selected by repetition of some stimulus that had previously altered the probabilities of responses of other cell groups.

Group-Degenerate Selection in the Brain

With this background, we can now specify in more detail the system of group-degenerate selection that we suppose to have been evolved for higher brain functions. To begin with, the discussion will be limited to cortical areas, the thalamus, and the limbic system; the function of other parts of the neuraxis can then be considered in perspective.

The first question of importance is: What does the CNS recognize?—that is, what is the elementary substrate for higher brain function? Beyond the level of the interaction of an outside signal with sensory receptors, which can operate in a linear or nonlinear fashion (Mountcastle, 1957, 1967), the assumption here will be that the substrates for recognition are the spatiotemporal patterns of spikes and graded potentials (and their chemical concomitants) occurring in *groups of neurons*. By *recognition* I mean the selective and characteristic discriminative response of one or more groups of neurons to such patterns initiated or present in other groups to which they have access. The response of such recognizing groups is manifested in alterations in their further patterns of firing and in stable or metastable synaptic changes. A theoretical account of the possible internal properties of neuronal groups, on which recognition between groups might be based, has been given by Wilson and Cowan (1973). It is important to stress that the present assumptions do not exclude recognition of the state of a single neuron in a hierarchy. In general, however, the patterns recognized by cell groups are assumed to be those generated by other groups. Some support for this position is obtained from the studies of Hubel and Wiesel (1974) on feature detection in the striate cortex and associated areas.

Although the neuroanatomical evidence for cell groups in other regions is sparse, it may be useful for clarity to review more extensively the notions of cell group, repertoire, and recognition against the background of previous analyses (Bullock, 1961). A cell group is considered to be a collection of contiguous neurons whose intrinsic connectivity is defined by events in ontogeny and development. The connections within a group are not random but are definite. Each such group may have divergent or convergent extrinsic connections to and from other such groups; these connections are also neuroanatomically defined and nonrandom. According to this notion, although a single neuron can rarely serve as a "group," randomly connected nets are excluded (Bullock, 1961). In accord with the distinctions made by Bullock (1961), a group could constitute a multiple-input metastable feedback loop consisting of a definitely specified meshwork of mutually interacting neurons. But several additional properties of groups are assumed here that have not been assumed by previous theorists (Bullock, 1961; Grüsser and Grüsser-Cornehls, 1976).

   One of the most important is that groups form repertoires, that is, collections with diverse intrinsic connectivities but similar extrinsic connectivities. Such repertoires are prespecified during ontogeny and development and are degenerate with respect to recognition. Each group in a repertoire can act as a recognition unit carrying out one or more functions: encoding, decoding, identifying one of the lines of its extrinsic connectivity, timing signals, determining their strength or their rate of development or duration—all of which may be properties of signals from other cell groups. Of course, in most individual cases, the exact neural code is presently unknown.

   If the extrinsic connectivity of a group is divergent, leading to many other groups, then the output of the group may poll the other groups more or less effectively depending upon a variety of factors such as signal pattern, signal strength, and local inhibition. As in the case of a jury, these groups may or may not respond characteristically to the input from the first group. If the extrinsic connectivity is convergent upon a group, a variety of responses may occur, including facilitation, differences in timing, or different response patterns, all depending upon the location and properties of the extrinsic connections. Thus a group can have different portals for input, and input to different combinations of these portals may or may not influence its response. Because of its patterns of intrinsic and extrinsic connectivity, a group has available to its neurons a variety of modes of interaction with external signals. In any event, each group is not pluripotent—rather, it has a limited set of characteristic spatiotemporal response patterns of firing as well as a characteristic set of connections to other groups.

Among the variabilities offered by such a set of connections, the most important in determining higher-order functions is that offered by the opportunity to alter intrinsic connectivity plastically at synapses ("commitment"), leading to stabilization of a particular output pattern. This will be discussed later in detail. The main point here is that alterations of this type, occurring mainly in the intrinsic synapses, would lead to favoring of certain intrinsic connectivities over others.

We may now consider a hierarchy of responses that, in its later stages, will be nonlinear because of the presence of feedback and feedforward loops with their associated alterations of temporal patterns and response times. Ignoring this nonlinearity for the moment, we consider the hierarchy

$$S \longrightarrow R \longrightarrow (R \text{ of } R)_n, \quad n = 1, 2, 3, \ldots,$$

where S represents transduced sensory input from the environment (as but one example of input), R represents cortical cellular groups that can act as "recognizers" of that input (for example, groups of complex neurons in the striate cortex), and $(R \text{ of } R)$ represents groups of neurons in association cortex, or in temporal, frontal, or prefrontal cortex, that act as "recognizers of recognizers." According to this hierarchy, signals from neuronal groups of R (for example, a column) can be recognized by groups in $(R \text{ of } R)$. But it must be emphasized that at this higher level of recognition, the candidate neuronal groups in $(R \text{ of } R)$ form only a degenerate subset of all $(R \text{ of } R)$ cell groups (Figure 4a). That is, there is more than one group in $(R \text{ of } R)$ that can recognize a particular group in R; the response is based on the possibility of divergence and on multiple degenerate representation, providing together for the adequate recognition of R groups by the $(R \text{ of } R)$ repertoire. Note also that the arrows in this scheme do not necessarily imply unidirectional flow of information, but merely an initial sequence for recognition events. Indeed, the scheme must not be considered as strictly or exclusively hierarchical. Parallel organization is obviously of equal importance since it makes possible the output to action (motor response, neurohumoral response) from any level. The scheme also assumes that general properties of the input can be recognized early in the sequence $S{\to}R{\to}(R \text{ of } R)$.

We may summarize at this point by saying, somewhat loosely, that beyond the level of sensory transduction and sensory processing,

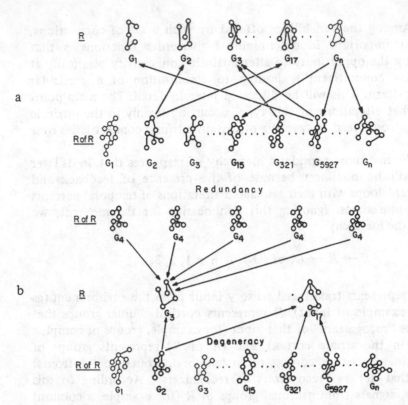

Figure 4. Interactions of degenerate groups in two repertoires, R and $(R$ of $R)$. Arrows connecting groups indicate recognition but do not necessarily imply unidirectional flow of information. (a) Degenerate recognition emphasizing bidirectional many–one relationships. (b) Contrast between redundancy and degeneracy in $(R$ of $R)$. Increase of redundant elements can only increase efficiency; for example, because of its structure and function, G_4, a strictly redundant group of $(R$ of $R)$, can never recognize G_{17} in R.

the CNS recognizes *modes of itself* selectively and in a nonlinear and degenerate fashion. It is revealing to ask whether such degenerate recognition could be successfully accomplished by isomorphic or strictly redundant cell groups in $(R$ of $R)$. Provided that the threshold requirement for recognition does not imply absolute specificity, but only distinctions among classes of similar patterns, the answer is no for the reasons adduced in the previous section (Figure 4b). Instead, a significant number of different but isofunctional cell groups, any one of which can respond to the class of patterns in R, is required. This implies that the same pattern can be recognized in more than one way and, indeed, that in successive presentations of the same pattern, different combinations of cell groups (R of R) would respond. Furthermore, there is no need to assume a priori that such groups necessarily have similar numbers or types of neurons.

Such a picture of neuronal groups selected from a degenerate repertoire must be distinguished from that of a fixed pattern of preprogrammed response that might occur in a single ganglion, and also from simple redundancy of neurons in subsystems such as the ganglia or nuclear cell masses in the brain. While these organizations are undoubtedly present in the brain, they cannot generate the kinds of responses produced by a degenerate repertoire.

So far I have only casually distinguished between the initial stable state and the ensuing responsive states of the subsets of cell groups in such a repertoire. According to the theory, the repertoire just described can be considered a *primary repertoire* formed during ontogeny and early development as a consequence of differentiation events leading to synaptic connectivity, both locally and in long pathways. As pointed out earlier, however, unless some form of stable amplification (or inhibition) of the responses of cell groups could occur in this repertoire, there would be no possibility for alteration of its properties as a result of experienced input. It would merely fluctuate reversibly in its selective response with varying relaxation times. It is at this point that we must suppose that the selection of certain subgroups results in an alteration of the probability that these subgroups will be selected again upon a repeated presentation of a similar stimulus pattern. As mentioned previously, this is assumed to occur as a result of synaptic alteration of some or all cells in a group so that intrinsic or extrinsic connectivity is functionally altered. This would be expected to occur mainly within the intrinsic connectivity of a group, with a concomitant change in its transfer functions, for example. The probability of selection could be decreased (inhibition) or increased (excitation, facilitation). In either case, a sufficient repetition of input within a given time is assumed to alter the likelihood of future selections of certain previously selected subgroups over their neighbors, a process that produces a *secondary repertoire*. Thus a secondary repertoire is a collection of different higher-order neuronal groups whose internal or external synaptic function has been altered by selection and commitment during experience. Moreover, repetition of input need not be confined to external signals, but may include reentrant inputs from the brain itself.

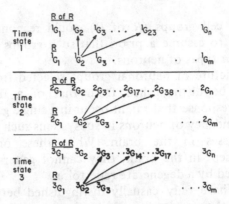

Figure 5. Variation of degenerate recognition with time depending upon polling and range of repertoires. Commitment or stable synaptic alteration of cells in (R of R) groups (indicated by a heavy arrow) occurs after repetition of recognition in different time states. Commitment is reflected in the increased probability of a subsequent response by certain groups in R. Superscripts on groups identify successive time states.

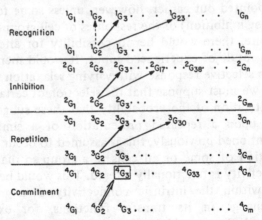

Figure 6. Fixation of responses in a degenerate network by a combination of discriminatory inhibition and commitment, raising the probability of response and leading to entrance of (R of R) group G_3 into a secondary repertoire as marked by the box. Dashed line: weak recognition. Solid line: good recognition. Thick line: excellent recognition. Double line: commitment.

One might visualize such a nonlinear, many–one, time-dependent, and degenerate response in the fashion shown in Figure 5, where the superscripts refer to the successive patterned states and the subscripts refer to different cell groups in the repertoire. An enhanced probability of positive or negative selection is represented in the figure by a heavy arrow.

Alteration of this probability may also be connected with the threshold for recognition events. Cell groups with higher repetition rates of response may, because they have a better "fit" with input, be stabilized more effectively. This may be achieved intrinsically, but more likely by means of escape from inhibition. At the same time, an inhibitory signal that suppressed some recognizing cell groups having less response to the original input would effectively sharpen the specificity of the overall response and also enhance its stabilization. Thus cell group selection may occur in a filtered fashion—first by stimulation of groups that react more or less well and then by inhibition (or competitive exclusion) of those selected groups with an insufficient response in relation to some threshold (Figure 6).

We may now ask about the overall properties of such a system and then consider the evidence for the existence of candidate cell groups having such properties. Obviously the alterations of selective probabilities represent a memory phenomenon; what has not been emphasized in Figure 6 is the associative nature of this memory (Longuet-Higgins, Willshaw, and Berneman, 1970) that results from the properties of degenerate selection. In a later section, this will be extensively discussed in connection with the conditions for consciousness. A brief consideration of associative memory in degenerate systems may serve here to set the stage for that discussion.

Association involves an ordering such that presentation in input of various attributes of an object results in a linkage between these attributes in output (Figure 7). A whole group of such orderings in storage can form an associative memory if the means of access and readout are available. In the ideal case, presentation in the proper context of any one of a set of stored items in an input should elicit recall of part or all of that set. Under certain conditions, related items

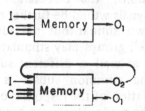

Figure 7. Representation of an associative memory in which input patterns I (for example signals from cell groups) in a context C (representing background, inhibition, or other patterns) results in related output patterns O. Output patterns such as O_2 may be reentered as input in such a system.

Gerald M. Edelman

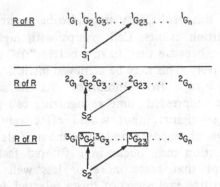

Figure 8. Association resulting from degenerate recognition and commitment for two unrelated signals S_1 and S_2. Heavy and light arrows indicate degree of recognition. Groups in squares are committed to secondary repertoire.

not in that set should also be able to elicit that recall. In the brain, it is likely that this type of storage is content-addressable and that access is simultaneous and parallel.

A degenerate collection of cell groups has a number of features that could lead to association and yield a memory with such properties. Certain neuronal groups may recognize a given signal pattern only more or less well. Indeed, some of these groups may be capable of recognizing some other signal pattern better than the one to which they have responded in a particular event. This raises the possibility that two different events may elicit responses from the same group as well as simultaneously eliciting responses from completely different groups (Figure 8). Moreover, if the probability of response of all of these groups is altered by multiple presentations, there is an increased likelihood of their being excited together on future presentations of either signal event. Inasmuch as these groups may have different neuroanatomical connections, the association with other groups responding to additional signals would be further enhanced.

Presentation of two similar but not identical patterns to a degenerate collection of cell groups may stimulate a common subset of groups in that collection as well as different subsets unique to each pattern (Figure 9). If the common subset is connected to other neuronal groups, an association of the responses of those groups to that of the shared subset can be made. Moreover, sequential presentation of two related patterns can elicit the same responses by activating that subset, and (R of R) groups reading any of the subsets may thus become associated.

There is the additional possibility that recognition of a cell group pattern requires only part of the intrinsically connected neuronal

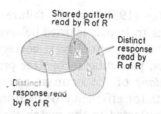

Shared pattern
read by R of R

Distinct
response
read by
R of R

Distinct
response read
by R of R

Figure 9. Reading, with association, of different collections of groups elicited by a structurally similar pair of input patterns, *a* and *b*. Collections of cell groups recognizing the patterns are marked by *a* and *b*; the shared subset of responding groups is marked by *x*. Different (*R* of *R*) groups reading these patterns may become associated in their responses.

set within the recognizing group, leaving another part free for other recognitions. This is a special case akin to recognition by two spatially different groups. But because of local connectivity, it raises further opportunities for particular kinds of association by recombination of features within a group.

In discussing association, we must also consider the degree of hierarchical nesting possible in selective recognition events in associative systems of this kind. By *nesting* I mean the number of successive recognitions across different levels of organization such as *R* and (*R* of *R*). Although nested recognition can occur, the scheme has no implicit or necessary hierarchical restriction. An (*R* of *R*) subgroup can selectively "recognize" another (*R* of *R*) subgroup; recognition is not limited to cell groups of another level, such as *R*. This leads to the possibility of a reading *of* the states of cell groups whose probability of response has been stably altered in previous selections *by* cell groups that have not been so altered. In view of the degenerate nature of the repertoire, it also implies that a given pattern can be "stored" in the response of several and perhaps many isofunctional but not necessarily isomorphic groups. This provides ample opportunity for associative interactions in the reflexive recognition of (*R* of *R*) groups. At the same time, however, it must be stressed that certain neuronal groups must always remain in the primary repertoire. Indeed, there may have to be some neurons that are incapable of commitment so that groups of which they are composed do not become fixed to a given pattern of response.

Another important general feature of a system of group-degenerate selection is its *distributive property*. A particular stable selected state or response to an input pattern is not likely to be uniquely represented in only one cell group in one place. Indeed, beyond particular neuroanatomical restrictions, there is no requirement that selected isofunctional cell groups be contiguous. This is in accord with the observations of Lashley (1950) on the failure of transection and ablation of cortical regions to impair learned behaviors, but it does not imply that his notion of equipotentiality is correct. Indeed, one can imagine that in some cases, particular recognizer properties are present only in certain larger *regions* of the brain as a result of evolutionary selection and requirements for efficiency of neuronal communication. This would appear to be reflected in the match that is found between the functional adaptation and density of peripheral innervation and the amount and sophistication of the central representation linked to that periphery. This qualified picture of distributed neuronal groups is consistent with evidence for gross localization of function but is still in accord with the distribution of both memory and learning patterns. It is also consistent with the functional interaction of distant groups to yield complex brain functions, as detected after brain lesions and ablation experiments (Luria, 1973). There is evidence for great variation in the threshold for tolerance of tissue destruction of different cell groups (Russell and Espir, 1961), a fact also in accord with group-degenerate selection.

It is important to emphasize that in a selective system, degeneracy and diversity are more important than absolute repertoire size. The requirement for limiting large numbers of diverse cell groups in a degenerate repertoire (see Figure 1) is nonetheless consistent with the failure to find neuronal types that are radically different from normal in nanocephalics (Seckel, 1950) and the failure to correlate higher function with gross estimates of brain size. Below a certain number of cells, however, and in the absence of the opportunity to make certain synaptic connections, the repertoire would fail either to contain sufficiently degenerate subsets or to be polled by input patterns in an efficient manner.

Neither the distributive nor the associative property is unique to selective systems; various instructive models that have these properties have been proposed (Longuet-Higgins, Willshaw, and Berneman, 1970; Cooper, 1973). The group-degenerate selection model places more emphasis on the features of cell groups and less on the general properties of an overall network, however. Thus it strongly emphasizes the role of neuroanatomy and development as fundamental in constructing particular primary repertoires and particular kinds of connected cell groups.

It is important to stress how the notion of memory is altered by the concept of group-degenerate selection. Fixation of the responses of a cell within a group or of the whole group via several cells can alter selective patterns at any level of recognition. In terms of group-degenerate selection, memory is not a localized property of any particular region of the nervous system. Rather, it is a general reflection of the enhanced interaction of cell groups that contain selectively committed cells and their synapses. If one adds to this the possibilities of long-tract connectivity, the notion of an active storage with high associative power, and the concept of reentrant signaling to be discussed below, there is no need to posit memory as a property of a given region or as an exclusive emergent property of some particular higher brain function. Whatever the microscopic or molecular mechanism of memory or cell interaction (for example, new dendritic connections, metastable membrane and cell surface changes in dendritic spines, molecular alterations of synapses), this property is an obligate consequence of group-degenerate selection and must therefore be a property of neurons as they function in cell groups. Memory readout is not posed as a special problem; the *process* does not differ from other forms of neuronal communication in the group-degenerate system.

What can we say about the neuronal substrate for repertoire degeneracy? There is an emerging realization that in higher brain centers such as the olfactory bulb (Shepherd, 1972), the law of dynamic polarity associated with the classical neuron doctrine fails. Instead, the picture of a highly diverse set of dendritodendritic, axodendritic, axosomatic, and dendritosomatic connectivities emerges. This picture is likely to be seen in other cortical regions, and together with the evidence of Golgi II neuron interactions, and the impressive increase in the number of LCNs during phylogeny and in ascending the neuraxis (Rakic, 1975), it suggests an anatomical view entirely consistent with group-degenerate selection. The development of the neocortex appears to have been accomplished by a large increase in the number of cell columns or units as well as in their interconnections. In addition to the anatomy of cortical areas (Chow and Leiman, 1970; Peters, Paley, and Webster, 1976), that of certain limbic and reticular formation areas (Isaacson and Pribram, 1975a) is also consistent with the features of a degenerate repertoire.

While repertoires of cell groups are not random, there is a large opportunity for individual variation in different regions and in different individual brains. Nevertheless, according to the theory, different brains should be able to carry out a particular recognition event with equal effectiveness even though, in their functional history, different isofunc-

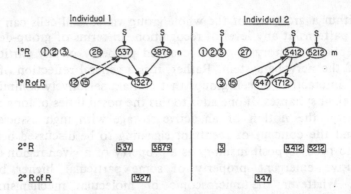

Figure 10. An illustration of the individuality of trace information during establishment of a secondary repertoire in different individuals given similar primary repertoires. Trace formation on differing neuroanatomical backgrounds could alter the encounter frequencies of cell groups represented by different numbers in different individuals. $1°R$ and $2°R$ denote primary and secondary recognizer repertoires; a similar notation is used for $(R$ of $R)$ repertoires.

tional subgroups were selected (Figure 10). The consequence of the presence of degeneracy is therefore a high degree of diversity and individuality. This provides for rare or unusual fluctuations in the neural repertoires of certain individuals.

According to the present theory, embryogenesis and development provide a first repertoire; early learning and selective interactions lead to development of a second repertoire via chemical facilitation and memory processes. After several selective events, the statistics of the primary repertoire are altered so that a secondary repertoire of selected cell groups emerges. Although the statistics of repertoire response are thereby altered, a large number of possibilities still remain open. Cell groups in this secondary repertoire would, in general, have a higher likelihood of undergoing repeated selection by similar inputs than would isofunctional groups in the primary repertoire. It must be emphasized, however, that this is only a probabilistic statement; upon repeated presentation of a signal, groups in the primary repertoire could still undergo selection in preference to those in the secondary repertoire in response to a variety of circumstances. In any case, for a given input pattern at any time, primary repertoire groups capable of specific recognition of a given signal would still far outnumber those in the secondary repertoire. But because of the previous operation of commitment and thresholding events, not many would be as "sharply tuned" to that signal.

The central neural construct is thus considered to be a result of two different selective processes: ontogenetic development of the first repertoire and selection by environmental interaction to form a second repertoire. The relationships of transition periods and critical periods in both processes—such as those explored by Blakemore (Blakemore and Van Sluyters, 1974) for Hubel and Wiesel neurons and by Piaget (1950, 1954) in the psychology of early growth and development—deserve extensive investigation in terms of these concepts.

Later I shall make some specific comments concerning the embryogenesis of the first repertoire. At this point, it may be more pertinent to summarize the process of second repertoire formation. This process leads to formation of a unique trace of selection events, to an enhancement of the probability of reselection of elements of the second repertoire over those of the first, and to alterations of likelihoods of encounter thresholds, possibly at synapses. In such a system, the order of development of the second repertoire is very important. The number of cell groups, the number of cells, and the number of synapses possible in the CNS make for an extraordinarily large number of possibilities in forming a second repertoire. Regardless of the number of selective events, however, there would still remain a large, indeed a major, pool of uncommited cell groups in the first repertoire.

The foregoing analysis bears on two key statements of Mountcastle (1976): "The central problem for brain physiology is how to understand the actions of large populations of neurons, actions that may not be wholly predictable from properties of subsets" and "The central problem of the intrinsic physiology of the cerebral cortex is to discover the nature of neuronal processing within the translaminar chains of interconnected cells (in columns)." In the light of the analysis so far, these statements might be transformed as follows: *The main problem of brain physiology is to understand the nature of repertoire building by populations of cell groups.* Of course, the solution of this problem requires a knowledge of transmission, polling, and encounter and of amplification and stabilization of synaptic events at the molecular level. The present theory is phenomenological in the sense that, at the level of description attempted here, it does not depend upon specification of these processes in great detail. This does not gainsay the need for an exact understanding of these processes; it simply stresses that a variety of different solutions would be compatible with group-degenerate selection.

Reentrant Selective Signaling
and the Neural Substrates for Consciousness

So far this discussion of the degenerate selection of cell groups has ignored specific circuits of neuronal connections and their relation to particular higher brain functions. The task I shall undertake here is to consider the central problem of consciousness and to show how degenerate selection and cell group signaling in a reentrant fashion can provide the necessary conditions for an explanation of this phenomenon at the cellular level. The problem of consciousness has resisted analysis in an experimental context until recently, and it still remains a formidable challenge. Perhaps no other subject has gathered around it so varied a set of speculations as consciousness: the mind-body problem (Campbell, 1970), the existence of spirits, the evaporation of the notion of "mind" by semantic analysis (Ryle, 1949), and the possibility of a pontifical neuron (Sherrington, 1941). Clearly there is a collective opinion that this brain function is somehow the central one that must be understood for a complete insight into learning and other higher functions.

Fortunately there are now some developments that allow us to narrow the issue. The experiments of Penfield (1975), Jasper (1966), and others (Isaacson and Pribram, 1975b) on the role of the reticular formation in arousal indicate that there are areas of the brain outside of the cortex that are necessary for consciousness. On the other hand, the experiments of Sperry (1970a) demonstrate that there are separate and specific hemispheric localizations of different brain functions related to consciousness. In addition, there is evidence that the hippocampal and limbic systems can function to distinguish novelty and read out short-term memory in a fashion that might modulate input to the conscious brain (Vinogradova, 1975). Perhaps the main impact of this and related work is that consciousness is *not* a property of the entire brain, but rather is a result of *processes* occurring in certain defined areas (admittedly gross), for example, the two cortical hemispheres, the thalamocortical radiations (Mountcastle, 1974), and the limbic and reticular systems. Nevertheless, the kinds of interactions that lead to consciousness remain unspecified.

The question therefore is: What are these interactions and what properties would they be expected to have? In attempting to answer this question, any proposed hypothesis obviously must not violate the laws of thermodynamics, posit entities that cannot be measured, or lead to an infinite regression of specified temporal recognition events. On the positive side, it must stress the main dynamic function of the brain in mediating between experience and action. In so doing, it must be able to account for updating of past storage and for the temporal properties of recall. Can any general model that includes group-degenerate selection be constructed that would meet these restrictions and account for a temporal sequence of conscious and recall states, the need for updating an informational store (MacKay, 1970), and the differentiation of immediate and long-term experience? And at its limit, could such a model be consistent with the distinction between self and nonself?

Among other things, such a model must specifically account for the continuity of perception, for temporal succession, and for the detection of novelty. The first decision to be made in building this model is whether to adopt a continuous or a discontinuous temporal mode of information processing. There are several reasons for choosing a discontinuous mode: (1) processing of any event must occur before awareness of it (that is, some output must be prepared before the outcome of a sensory input is decided); (2) there are stringent temporal constraints on recall that require the operation of a real-time clock; and (3) as discussed below, a discontinuous mode greatly simplifies our understanding of how coding for spatiotemporal continuity can occur in a degenerate selective system. These and other considerations to be discussed below suggest that the elementary processes leading to consciousness may be phasic, that is, they may require cyclic repetition of a sequence of neuronal events.

An approach to constructing a phasic model is illustrated in Figure 11. Suppose that some cell group in R receives sensory or

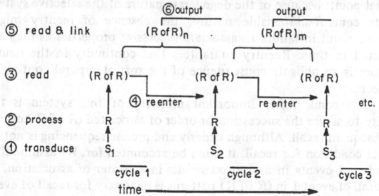

Figure 11. Reentrant signaling in the path from inputs S to recognizers R to "recognizers of recognizers" (R of R). The scheme indicates reentry in successive cycles; the temporal order of events within two successive cycles is indicated by numbers. The associative aspects of reentrant signaling are not indicated in this scheme (see Figure 12). $(R$ of $R)_n$ and $(R$ of $R)_m$ are higher-order associative neuronal groups whose output may reenter at later points, activate motor output, make associations, etc.

sensorimotor information and that its action and storage are recognized by several cell groups in (R of R). At the same time, suppose that the same sensory input to the limbic and reticular centers is processed and relayed by the thalamus to the cortex to stabilize these particular (R of R) groups for several immediately subsequent events. By *stabilization* or *fixation* I mean, in this context, the continued firing of these groups in their typical patterns. This constitutes the first temporal phase of a cycle of input processing. Now suppose that in the succeeding phase, this processed signal is reentered at a high level in the $S \to R \to (R$ of $R)$ information path of the next cycle. The reentered signal and new (R of R) signals from subsequent inputs are then read by (R of R) groups that make associations with stored patterns in (R of R) cell groups of the second repertoire as well as with groups in the first repertoire if there is any novelty. This constitutes the second or reentrant phase of input. Such a system is designed so that an internally generated signal is reentered *as if it were an external signal.* This is a key feature of the model, and it has two functions: to provide a means for dealing with novelty and to provide a match and a link between inner states and new sensory inputs of various modalities. In detail, it must be able to relate modalities as well as cross-correlate them. A possible means of accomplishing this will be described later.

As a result of reentry, this model assures that there will be continuity or linkage between successive phasic inputs. There is therefore no need for any higher-order recognition of the connection between states of objects as they are registered in time. This is an essential point: because of the degenerate nature of the selective system and its content-addressable nature, the absence of reentry might otherwise result in failure to associate successive properties as they are abstracted in time. Reentry guarantees that continuity in the neural construct is an obligate consequence of the spatiotemporal continuity of objects.

A second highly important property of this system is the capacity to assure the succession or order of associated (R of R) events for subsequent recall. Although orderly and precise sequencing is not an obligate condition for recall, it must be accounted for. We assume that the order of events in a context results in an order of association, so that recall of event 1 in (R of R) patterns is necessary for recall of event 2 and so on. The same "clock states" of the system required for the original integration and abstraction would then be used to call out this succession in the same measure and dimensions of real time. Obviously, however, the clock would only provide a real-time *base* for this process; recall need not take the same amount of time as the original events. The actual length of a reentrant cycle in real time will be discussed later.

Novelty of signals is dealt with in this system by comparison between reentrant and new signals in a cycle as well as by the fact that there are primary and secondary repertoires. Completely new information must activate primary repertoire. Match and mismatch of signal information may be accounted for by discriminating between activation of secondary repertoire and primary repertoire. The exact means by which the two repertoires are distinguished is not obvious, but frequency or latency properties may be sufficient to distinguish neuronal activity from each. The additional possibility that stored information in secondary repertoire is compared with new input in a highly efficient fashion to detect novelty cannot be neglected, however.

In the absence of a knowledge of the detailed anatomy, it is difficult to choose among the various circuits consistent with the scheme of reentrant signaling. But the theory does assume a certain minimal set of connections. Each afferent portal to the brain is linked first to a restricted set of R's located in the primary sensory cortex by connections that are mainly invariant. Divergance then occurs to (R of R) groups with greater or lesser specificity. The sensory signatures disappear at this point, and associative reentry leads to expression of higher functions by the many classes of (R of R) groups, which are no longer arranged sequentially. It is pertinent that the thalamocortical and corticothalamic radiations provide candidate circuits for portions of the reentry scheme (Mountcastle, 1974).

At this point, it is important to point out the conditions necessary for such a scheme to function and to describe some of its consequences. Assuming the proper anatomy for the moment, this scheme requires:

1. Recognition of R by (R of R) groups in temporal, frontal, and prefrontal regions. Under the scheme of selection, this is likely to involve neuronal divergence, rather than convergence, as a first step.

2. Pulsed states of input consistent with cerebral, thalamocortical, hippocampal, and limbic-reticular rhythms.

3. (R of R) subsets in secondary repertoire with stably altered synapses and transfer functions expressing committed patterns representing the storage of previous states.

4. Degenerate recognition of (R of R) cell groups by other (R of R) cell groups. At some level, convergence must also occur to provide an "abstract summary" or transform of complex patterns.

5. Stabilization of the selected (R of R) groups for at least one cycle (according to the present scheme, this is done via the limbic-reticular afferents in either a general or a specific fashion).

6. Short-term storage for holding patterns of "world inputs" (input state 1) and potentiality for storing reentrant "self inputs" (input state 2). Such storage allows for matching and association and is considered to be itself degenerate and widely distributed.

7. Linkage of (R of R) output to central states and to stored patterns concerned with the control of movement.

This model does not imply an infinite nest of recognizing neuronal groups. Indeed, since it depends upon comparisons between current input and stored states, and since associated degenerate groups are assumed to be available with similar recognition properties, it is not necessary that the same (R of R) cell group or groups recognize inputs in two successive cycles. The degeneracy of these groups would imply that the same input state could be recognized at different times by more than one such group. It is nevertheless important that *within* a cycle the same (R of R) groups be used, and a change of (R of R) groups must not interrupt the execution of a motor output pattern. As I shall describe in detail, awareness is considered to arise from the (R of R) repertoire having access to R and to stored multimodally generated states within itself. In turn, this access can lead to generation of associatively related signals, which are then processed again on the same input lines as an S signal; that is, the system is reentrant. The entire cycle provides for the possibility of modification by (R of R) output of the sensory input and its thresholds as well as for alteration of arousal and intentional or attentional states. The basic a priori condition for the conscious state is the ability to review the internal state by continual reentry of stored information. This review is obviously altered by the ability to recognize novelty and by states of arousal.

So far I have suggested that the conscious state requires the phasic recognition by degenerate (R of R) groups of signals representing the internal state of the organism and input. The discussion has centered on a rather artificial example of a single sensory signal of one modality. But it has not reemphasized a property of degenerate networks that is essential to their function in relation to conscious states: the associative nature of interactions among degenerate cell groups. Many of the neuronal cell groups called up by a given signal pattern match that pattern only more or less well. Moreover, these groups may contain neuronal configurations that can also recognize other, unrelated signal patterns more or less well: indeed, these other patterns might be recognized with even higher probabilities (or closer "fit") than the given pattern. This brings up the possibility that, because of their "unused" potential information, such cell groups have associative properties that allow them to interact with a variety of signals arising either from incoming information or from $(R \text{ of } R)$ store. Thus a cell group may be used more than once by different signals or may be used simultaneously by two signals. Evidence has in fact been obtained for multisensory input to a given cortical neuron (Eccles, 1966b), although this may be more concerned with level setting than with association.

The associative nature of the reentrant system would result in readout of groups of $(R \text{ of } R)$ neurons that represent past multimodal experiences. Indeed, one variant of the model (Figure 12) suggests that

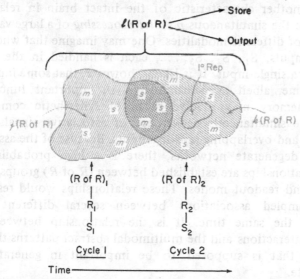

Figure 12. A diagram illustrating reentrant signals in two subsequent cycles to emphasize the associative multimodal readout of collections of groups containing stored patterns of past sensory inputs (s) or sensorimotor events (m). This readout is completed after the reentrant stage, thus linking the two successive patterns of $(R \text{ of } R)$ groups responding to R. Here $j(R \text{ of } R)$ and $k(R \text{ of } R)$ represent varying numbers of groups involved in the associative response to $(R \text{ of } R)_1$ and $(R \text{ of } R)_2$. The overlap of these groups (marked by the cross-hatched area) is related to similarities in S_1 and S_2. The area marked $1°\text{Rep}$ refers to the associative access to primary repertoire groups by new information contained in S_2. The $l(R \text{ of } R)$ neurons can store the result, output to other $(R \text{ of } R)$ groups, or call upon central routines for motor response. Continuity depends upon the linked reading of $(R \text{ of } R)_1$ and $(R \text{ of } R)_2$ and of the associative responses in $j(R \text{ of } R)$ and $k(R \text{ of } R)$. Novelty may be detected in part by differential response in the readout of neuronal groups in primary and secondary repertoires.

it is the readout of these groups in relation to current input that is essential for establishing the conscious state. Such associative properties raise the question of how the "correct" (R of R) groups in the store are made accessible for comparison with the output of R cell groups. One solution to this problem is to consider that the (R of R) groups that are in the secondary repertoire can recognize R states directly. This is possible if each such cell group has alternative configurations that allow responses to new signals in addition to those for which it was originally selected. A more specific (and I believe more attractive) alternative is that the (R of R) groups that recognize S via R also recognize the patterns of other (R of R) groups in storage. In any case, retrieval and comparison is not by means of random access; rather, it is related to a dense network of associative interactions that are enhanced in a degenerate system.

This associative potential may also be of importance in considering another characteristic of the intact brain in relation to consciousness: the simultaneous *parallel processing* of a large variety of input signals of different modalities. One may imagine that when there are several inputs, S_1, S_2, S_3, . . ., each is handled in the fashion described for a single input. It is likely, however, that some inputs will overlap in time, albeit asynchronously. An important function of associative memory may involve recall of synesthetic components related to the simultaneous occurrence of associative signals arising from parallel and overlapping sensory inputs. Because of the associative property of degenerate networks, there is a high probability that numerous relationships are established between (R of R) groups in both the storage and readout modes. These relationships would result in a series of sampled associations between several different signals occurring at the same time. It is the relationship between these multimodal interactions and the multimodal abstract patterns that have been stored that is supposed to be important in generating the conscious state.

Output to motor systems and reentrant input from store would provide continuous confirmation or alteration of this relationship. The presence of abstract representation, perhaps arising from convergence of afferent pathways on cell groups in those areas of cortex carrying out linguistic functions, would serve both to condense and to integrate past experiences. The cell groups serving such a function could be called upon to integrate conscious states arising from current input by associative interaction. All of these factors would tend to make the transient, probabilistic, parallel, and phasically distinct processes described previously connect in a richly associated network of interactions that is constantly changing under changes of input. In effect, this would smooth out and connect responses and patterns of awareness resulting from the activity of different (R of R) groups. It would also provide for rapid variable access to large portions of storage with new associations at each cycle. Moreover, as pointed out above, because the access to storage also depends on a cycle and "clock state," the formidable problem of generating a memory of time duration of a given set of recalled events is mitigated: the same time base is used for both recall and awareness.

If this analysis is correct, a subject would be aware of duration but would not be aware of alternate states in the cycle, because memory states, parallel processing of other signals, and asynchrony would lead to a smoothing of various inputs over longer time periods than a single reentrant cycle. This touches upon the critical question of the time period assumed for the phasic states. Hippocampal rhythms with frequencies of 3–8 Hz have been detected, and it is conceivable that cycles could be as long as 300 msec. There is, however, no clear-cut correlation between informational processing and θ rhythms (Dennett, 1975). Perhaps more detailed information on the temporal interactions of the thalamic pacemaker with the ascending reticular system will provide the most relevant information (Mountcastle, 1974). The evidence for a minimal "activation period" of about 200–500 msec for awareness of a near-threshold stimulus is also pertinent (Libet, 1966). I would suspect that much faster entry is possible; work in experimental psychology suggests that a full perception requires no more than 100 msec of intracortical processing time. One calculation that might be valuable would be to estimate the transmission time and delay expected in all parts of the cycle postulated here, but at present, in the absence of detailed anatomical information, this calculation is not possible. It is worth noting, however, that after periods of time of this order of magnitude, the hippocampus experiences inhibitory signals and "wipe-out" (Pribram and Isaacson, 1975). This is just what would be required in portions of a phasic reentrant scheme. Moreover, the existence of a short-term memory of the kind known to be related to hippocampal transactions (Vinogradova, 1975) may also be essential to "sample and hold" phasic input for the high-level processing described here.

In dealing with novelty, the brain is centrally concerned with mediating between experience and action. Because the brain functions for action, it may seem strange that the discussion here has not centered upon motor output or function. Evaluation of the evidence (Evarts et al., 1971) that central programming of motor patterns is apparently predominant over simple reflex patterns enables us, however, to took upon motor repertoire in much the same fashion as sensory repertoire. An important feature to be stressed is that central states can selectively call for whole patterns of motor activity that have been previously shaped by selective processes. Furthermore, there is evidence (Vanderwolf et al., 1975) that hippocampal function in attentional states is related to the performance of motor acts.

There is one particularly important feature of sensorimotor interaction that focuses on the input to a selective system: the motor repertoire further channels, restricts, and helps to program encounters in the sensory domain. Carrying out certain motor acts may therefore alter the density and nature of input signals and help to refine selection in ways that would otherwise not be very probable. The influence of motor functions on the paradigms for conscious behavior has been discussed penetratingly by MacKay (1966).

To summarize, it may be valuable to reconsider, at a naive level, the minimal set of features that are absolutely required for awareness according to the reentrant-signal model. There must be degenerate selection, reflexive recognition of (R of R) neuronal groups by each other, (R of R) storage, processing of activation and S signals in a coordinate fashion, rhythmic activity with phased states, and appropriate signal-holding networks to allow reentrant processing and coordination with external sensory input for at least some short period of time. Removal of higher midbrain input, removal of (R of R) storage, and removal of sensory input would each be expected to cause vast disturbances in consciousness. Clearly, however, after some time, this system would not be rigorously stimulus-bound: memory states and proprioceptive inputs could keep it functioning, if only in a deranged fashion (Jasper, 1966). One must conceive of (R of R) store as being kept in a continuously active state. Of course, alteration or obliteration of the phasic excitatory and inhibitory signals for alternate reentrant processing would also have massive effects. Indeed, one amusing prediction of this model is that consciousness is "digitized" and lagged: input state 1 is a period in which *no* consciousness of the signal state is yet possible. A test within the time period of this state, if feasible, would reveal no awareness of signal content. Only in input state 2 is there the possibility of "consciousness."

The Sufficient Conditions for Conscious Awareness

The discussion has not yet dealt with all the sufficient conditions for awareness, nor has it considered the related problem of the quality of sensory modalities. At a certain point, the problem of quality is private and not scientifically testable. At best, public verifications can occur by means of reports, but the direct comparison of sensory qualities identically reported by two individuals still cannot verify their qualitative similarity or difference. This is all the more true if one takes into account the richly different present phenomenal states of two conscious reporters. But there is some profit in considering certain aspects of sensory quality in the light of a selective theory of brain function.

To begin with, it is useful to note that, because sensory modalities are mediated by signals on "labeled lines," there is no problem in principle of identifying *different* modalities. Their recognition by R and (R of R) groups proceeds, however, through a series of hierarchically ordered abstract transforms that result from the activity of these groups. According to the selective theory, simultaneity of inputs $S_1, S_2, \ldots, S_n$ is sufficient to raise the possibility of higher-order associations among their respective transforms; it is not necessary that these S's be causally connected.

With this in mind, it is likely that the sufficient conditions for awareness arise from a historical process in each individual whereby increasingly abstract routines are placed in the secondary repertoire. The additional possibility must be entertained, however, that *early* associations with those areas of the brain concerned with affective states are critical in distributing into storage a series of response patterns that are sampled frequently later in life. These distributed "primitives" may consist of modally related patterns of motor and sensory responses that have been initially mediated, for example, by hypothalamic areas and the medial forebrain bundle. Such patterns may lead to chemically mediated changes in a variety of somatic responses. Although their "quality" is not discussable in scientific terms because the only possible access to these responses is indirect (behavioral observation) or verbal (possibly at a time when verbal communication has not yet developed), later verbally reportable "qualities" may be tied to their responses by abstraction through (R of R) groups. The capacity to distinguish modalities may play a major role in this process inasmuch as associative cross-correlations of modalities are made by the simul-

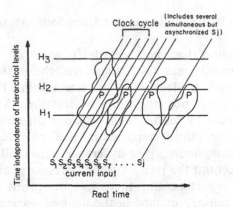

Figure 13. An attempt to illustrate how successive cycles of phasic reentry with associative readout may call upon hierarchical levels of (R of R) neurons of increasing degrees of abstract coding. "Primitives" (P), consisting of distributed stored patterns of early experiences associated to various extents with different hierarchical levels $H_1 - H_3$, have a high likelihood of interaction with current input and of being read by (R of R) neurons. The three arbitrarily chosen hierarchical levels of storage consist of (R of R) neuronal groups that contain increasingly abstract information, and they therefore represent a variety of routines accumulated during experience. The higher levels contain more abstract stable representations that do not depend as much on immediate temporal change. For example, H_1 might represent instantaneous feature detection and pattern recognition; H_2, associative and perceptual routines; and H_3, internal models or "theories" of self, possibly based in linguistic routines. Association of current input S_j at H_1 and H_2 leading to modality correlation may be read by groups that associate with H_3. Time relations, modality, and affective connections may lead to different motor responses dependent upon access to primitives.

taneity of different S inputs. In any event, the expression of sensory quality is a highly abstract process, as pointed out by Miller and Johnson-Laird (1976). In view of the evidence from a variety of studies (Piaget, 1950, 1954; Miller and Johnson-Laird, 1976), this also implies that *awareness* of quality is a historically developed process.

Figure 13 illustrates the later access to various (R of R) hierarchies via cross-correlation of S's and interaction with primitives in the repertoire. Because of the complexity of these interactions, this diagram and the assumptions upon which it is based must both be taken as skeletal and highly provisional.

From this discussion, it is clear that if one insists that the sufficient conditions for consciousness must include an explanation of quality in the sense that it is experienced by an individual through direct acquaintance, then no scientific theory can be constructed that is satisfactory. The present theory has therefore not provided a definition of consciousness that would meet sufficiency conditions of the kind prescribed by philosophers. It can be said, however, that several previously annoying conditions have been removed by the present model:

1. The need for a "thinking homunculus" is removed by the ties between phasic reentrant processing and abstract multidimensional store, defining "self" and a world model in terms of past sensory and motor experience. In their most sophisticated forms, such models are likely to require the existence of elements capable of language (Miller and Johnson-Laird, 1976), but language is probably not generally necessary for their manifestation.

2. The need for an infinite regress or hierarchy is removed by the degeneracy and associative properties of cell groups. It is further relieved by the phasic reentrant nature of signaling, which allows "restarts" to occur without loss of reference to long-term memory. The divergent (degenerate) and convergent (abstracting) properties of (R of R) ensembles suggest that a *sequential* process can deal with nests of higher-ordered abstractions. Furthermore, because of the associative properties of group-degenerate selection, the need for a program or a "programmer" is mitigated. In this sense, the analogy between the higher nervous system and computers fails, although at higher levels such a system is capable of carrying out routines (Miller and Johnson-Laird, 1976).

3. No causal requirements are placed on input signals: simultaneity is sufficient, provided the time constants of cerebral, reticular, and limbic responses are met.

According to this view, conscious awareness requires temporal processes that are both parallel and sequential. There is a constant shuttling among cross-correlated multimodal signals, phasically accessing a historically developed storage. In the operational sense, this view states that if a machine with these properties were built, it would report conscious states (or reveal them under test). But the quality "by acquaintance" of its sensation or perception would be neither directly accessible nor operationally definable, unless the machine could be connected to a human nervous system, an even more unlikely event than the construction of the machine itself. About such qualities the machine might say, "If they were not this way, they would be that way." The main requirement for adequate functioning is that, having once labeled modalities, the machine must not confuse them.

Some Implications and Comparisons with Alternative Views

Some of the general implications of this model need to be stressed. First, there is no need to postulate that the molecules of the brain are *directly* influenced by conscious processes, as specified by

Sperry (1969, 1970b) in his proposals for modified mentalism. Besides being stated in terms that are thermodynamically unclear or dubious, such assumptions are unnecessary, as are emphases on emergent properties of "the brain" and holistic explanations without mechanistic detail. Under the present scheme, there is also no need to assume dualistic or pluralistic models (Eccles, 1974; Popper, 1974) or to rely upon determinate sequential states with psychophysical parallelism. Instead, the position taken here is consistent in the main with that of so-called central-state materialism (Campbell, 1970) or the more sophisticated versions of the "identity" hypothesis (Feigl, 1967). But as a scientific theory, the present argument proposes a particular set of mechanisms to account for higher brain function, and it must stand or fall on their verifiability, not upon its philosophical alliances.

It would be a mistake to conclude from the present description that a system of group-degenerate selection with reentry of signals operates in clockwork fashion. A slight fluctuation in the outside S signal, in activating systems, or in (R of R) would yield a very large number of isofunctional but nonidentical (R of R) responses to generating states from which further selective responses can occur. Selection can occur from cell groups participating in these states without "telling molecules what to do." At this level of description, the essential units of the conscious process are the cell groups, their connectivity, and the diverse repertoire they generate. Inasmuch as an enormous set of possibilities exists in comparing the states of such groups to successive states, particularly upon slight biasing of outside signals, there is no need to invoke determinate "mechanical" sequences of responses. This is all the more true if one considers that two equivalent states of consciousness may represent entirely different subsets of (R of R) repertoire. More important, recombination of such states would generate an almost limitless set of possibilities of association.

Given long-term memory in (R of R) and the ability to change the degree of processing of S and of activating signals, it is not particularly difficult to see how such a system could be modulated for planning and programming, for limiting S signals to proprioceptive inputs, or for emphasizing (R of R) interactions in altered attentional states (Vinogradova, 1975). In this connection, it is worth stressing again that the outcome at any time of the process occurring in a group-degenerate system with phasic reentry is probabilistically determined. For example, competitive selection between or among groups in the primary and secondary repertoires would be determined by (1) the polling process, that is, *which* cell group or groups of sufficient "fit" were first encountered by a given signal; (2) the presence of inhibitory processes that remove the responses of cell groups having lesser degrees of recognition; and (3) the degree of commitment and recognizing efficiency of a previously selected group in the secondary repertoire. This does not rule out the possibility in a mature system that S can be internally generated. Indeed, the replacement of or competition with an "external" S by an internally generated S would be essential for central planning and programming. But I suspect that this would require considerable prior selective experience and a higher-order processing that is related, in its most sophisticated forms, to the acquisition of language (Miller and Johnson-Laird, 1976). This holds a fortiori for refined distinctions between self and nonself (Piaget, 1950, 1954).

The main point in any case is that consciousness involves selective phasic interactions with both storage and external input, and that it depends absolutely upon both past and present experience. There is freedom ("free will" or "free agency") in such a system—the freedom is in the selective grammer of the neuronal groups—but this freedom is not limitless and is bound by a variety of constraints implicit in the properties of the neuronal groups.

Ontogeny and the Development of a First Repertoire

One of the major assumptions of the present theory is that prior to the development of conscious awareness (and essential for it) is the formation of a degenerate primary repertoire of recognizer cell groups. It is therefore essential to ask how such a first repertoire can develop during ontogeny and how its specific properties arose during evolution. At this point, I consider briefly the problem of ontogeny; in a later section, I shall make some comparative observations on the phylogeny of selective recognition systems.

The problem of embryogenesis, particularly of histotypic interactions, is at present far from solution at the molecular level. It is exquisitely posed by the development of higher nervous systems: for example, the "wiring problem" in developing a system such as the retinotectal projection is a formidable one (Barondes, 1976). One method of solving this problem essentially begs the question, namely, positing for each pair of cells a set of specific complementary recognizer molecules appearing under gene programming at the appropriate time of development (Moscona, 1974). An increasing body of evidence suggests, however, that such a prior repertoire of fixed gene products will not suffice. Both embryological (Hamburger, 1970) and regeneration (Weiss, 1970) experiments indicate, for example, that neuromuscular interactions are not prespecified but are modeled with time.

The data indicate that competitive exclusion of synapses occurs after initial multiple synapse formation, generally leading to 1:1 axon-to-muscle endplate ratios. Moreover, there is evidence that in the formation of some limb nerve plexuses, branching occurs before neuromuscular interaction (Landmesser and Pilar, 1970, 1972). In the optic tectum, removal of part of the tectum still allows formation of the proper gross projections (Yoon, 1975), suggesting that there is no prefixed code for *individual* cell–nerve fiber interaction. Finally, chemical analyses of retinal cell adhesion (Brackenbury et al., 1977; Thiery et al., 1977) implicate one or a few surface protein molecules but no extensive retina-specific or neuron-specific molecular repertoire.

The question therefore remains: How can a primary repertoire be formed? I shall suggest here the elements of a provisional hypothesis for the development of a primary repertoire whose properties are consistent with later group-degenerate selection to form a secondary repertoire.

1. Early in development, cell groups or polyclones are determined by gene expression and programming.

2. A large degeneracy is built into this system, there being many more cell groups than are ultimately used to make projections and connections. Many of the "unused" cells die (Prestige, 1970; Cowan, 1973).

3. A hierarchy of interactions occurs, with early decisions (such as branching of limb plexus neurons) being relatively few in number and decided by the gene program.

4. Interactions between cell groups are sequential, selective, and determined by mutual influence. For example, innervation of a limb by a portion of the spinal cord involves neuromuscular interactions and synapse formation, which depends upon anterograde and retrograde signals. Of the several synapses formed initially, usually only one survives. This selective survival of certain synapses is in accord with suggestions made by Weiss (1970) and by Changeux and Danchin (1976). The end result of such selective interaction is the loss of synap-

tic connections and the death of many CNS neurons during development. Nevertheless, after such selective stabilization (Changeux and Danchin, 1976), there remains a high degree of redundancy and degeneracy of specific isofunctional cell groups.

5. The major shaping of final connections at the level of synapses is therefore considered to be a selective interaction based on certain aspects of function. Once formed, these connections are in general not remade. Despite its selective nature, however, much in this system is still genetically predetermined, such as the position of the nuclei, their particular differentiation path, and their gross location. For example, ocular dominance columns are in general prespecified, but they can be committed during the critical period (Blakemore and Van Sluyters, 1974), and right and left eyes compete finally at the level of forming synapses with individual striate cortical neurons.

According to the present hypothesis, the first repertoire, like the second, is selectively formed at the level of its fine structure. But even if this view is correct, much has first to be done by gene programming, and the sequences of development are particularly critical (Bodian, 1970). The distinctive element in the hypothesis is that there is enormous degeneracy and selection early in the system, even before primary repertoire formation is complete. Later developments, such as those in critical periods, may reduce this degeneracy by selective synaptic stabilization (Changeux and Danchin, 1976). In ascending the neuraxis, one might expect later and later effects of critical selection and more and more evidence for degeneracy. There is very little need for degeneracy in certain subsystems, and evolutionary selection as well as critical-period shaping may remove it almost completely. But the need to develop a second repertoire in higher brain function requires that most of the degeneracy must remain in cortical and limbic-reticular areas. Under this view, the prefrontal, frontal, and temporal cortexes have a constantly extended critical period which in fortunate individuals may be delayed until death.

Evolution of Degenerate Systems, Cortex, and Local Circuit Neurons

There is ample evidence to indicate that in many nervous systems, no large need exists for degenerate repertoires. In insects (Bullock and Horridge, 1965) and molluscs (Kandel, 1976), for example, it is likely that the combination of fixed central pattern generators, unique but non-necessary neurons, compensatory behavioral options, and autonomous reflexes (Wilson, 1970) could all give rise to highly adaptive and complex forms of behavior without the kind of system discussed here. At some time during evolution, however, a new pattern of more plastic behavior must have had selective advantage. It is difficult to identify the origins of nervous systems capable of more refined learning, but it is likely (with the exception of higher developed marine organisms such as the octopus and the shark) that the major continuing developments occurred upon the assumption of terrestrial life by backboned organisms.

For certain species, survival under these conditions obviously involved a gradual shaping of eye, limb, and brain for the performance of complex sensorimotor acts. A more rapid change is seen in comparing the avian brain with that of mammals and primates: the shaping of cortical regions from external striatum (Nauta and Karten, 1970). And by the time of primate and hominid evolution, an extraordinarily rapid change occurred in the assumption of predominance of other neocortical regions over olfactory cortex. Consistent with the present theory, it appears likely that early awareness developed in step with both limbic (Vinogradova, 1975) and cortical change. The case for animal awareness in more modern forms has recently been eloquently made (Griffin, 1977); but the most striking case is still that of hominid development with its associated emergence of language and symbolic representation.

At the cellular level, neocortical development brought with it a large increase in the number of LCNs (Rakic, 1975; Schmitt, Dev and Smith, 1976). An emphasis on number alone (for example, a tenfold increase) does not serve, however, to suggest the massive increase in possible degenerate connectivity allowed by this development. According to the present theory, this and the associated increase in numbers of cell groups are the fundamental roots of higher-order consciousness with symbolic representation and awareness. While limbic-cortical and thalamocortical interactions and reentrant signaling may have already been developing slowly for purposes of behavioral advantages in mating, defense, or other fundamental mechanisms of survival, the emergence of a degenerate cortical repertoire mediated by extensive LCN connections was probably relatively explosive and marked a large selective advantage in CNS function.

If we assume, for the moment, that such developments in the CNS of "higher" mammals define a selective system, it is illuminating to compare its properties with those of two other biological systems known to involve selection: evolution and the immune system. Evolution is, of course, at the basis of all biology, and the immune system is a special development in the vertebrate species. If the present theory is correct, the cognitive systems that are realized most extensively in hominid brains constitute a third and most recent development (Table 1).

The first difference to note is the time scale of the selective operation: years to millions of years for natural selection, hours and days for immune selection, seconds and milliseconds for neural selection. The most "complicated" system is evolution, with hosts of conditions, species, and variations, among which is the appearence of the

TABLE 1
Some Characteristics of Selective Systems

	Evolution	Immune Response	Group Selection in CNS
Time scale for fixation of selective unit	Years to 10^6 years	Hours, days	Milliseconds, seconds, hours
Recency	3×10^9 years	600×10^6 years	?Birds (160×10^6 years) ?Mammals (200×10^6 years)
Overall system complexity	Greatest	Least	Median
Basis of variational process	Germ-line mutation	Somatic mutation	Somatic combination
Level of repertoire diversification	Mutation, gene flow	Somatic mutation of V genes	Embryogenesis, cell-group recombination
Unit of selection	Phenotype	Individual lymphocyte	Neuron and neuron group
Selective interactions	Environment (general) on phenotype by natural selection	Antigen and cell–cell interaction	Environment (sensory) via cell group–cell group interaction
Neutrality (neutral variants)	No	Yes	Yes
Renewal	Yes	Yes	No for cells Yes for synapses
Novelty	Yes	Rare or absent	Yes

brain itself. The next most complicated is the nervous system, with enormous numbers of cell types, abstract hierarchies, and selective interactions. The least complex is the immune system, with only one kind of target molecule (antibodies) and relatively few cell types.

In both the nervous system and immune systems, it is possible to have unused variants, and degeneracy in such somatic systems does in fact require the presence of many irrelevant neutral variants that will never be used. In the natural selection of organisms, however, there are few or no neutral mutations. Thus, although most surviving genomes are adaptively useful and viable in natural selection, in the CNS and in the immune system the patterns of selection are not necessarily adaptive.

What about "creativity" in such systems? Because of the limitation on input, clonal selection in immunity is a fixed system with variations on a theme; in natural selection and group-degenerate selection, completely new themes are possible. The immune system and evolution are renewable systems: new variants are always generated in the primary repertoire. In the CNS, this may not be true for cells but it may be true for synapses. From a methodological point of view, the problem of analysis of the two somatic systems of selection is different: in the immune system, much more is known about repertoire than about regulation; in the CNS, it is the other way around.

One final comment: If the higher brain is a selective system, it must be about as efficient a selective system as can be evolved, given the nature of the molecules that must be used. That is to say, the time constants of ionic fluxes and of impulse conduction and the neuronal packing are as efficient as can be arranged, and they result in a high signal-to-noise ratio and error-free propagation at extremely low thresholds. Encounter in the selective higher CNS is no problem; the problem is the development of powerful primary and secondary repertoires.

Some Predictions and Consequences

The main predictions of the group-degenerate theory are as follows:

1. Groups of cells, not single cells, are the main units of selection in higher brain function.

2. Such groups will be found to be multiply represented, degen-

erate, and isofunctionally overlapping. Many–one interactions via LCNs as well as via connecting axons will be found, with extensive divergence as a sign of degeneracy.

3. At the same time, multiple inputs from R and (R of R) neurons will be found to converge to the same (R of R) cell group, leading to abstract cell-group codes.

4. Although single neurons may occasionally function as a group, no pontifical neuron or single-neuron "decision unit" (Bullock, 1961) will ever be found at the highest levels of a system of any large degree of plasticity.

5. Selection will be found to play a large, but not exclusive, role in forming a first repertoire during embryogenesis. The position and occurrence of synapses is not determined by complementary inter-actions among surface proteins specific for each particular synapse. Thus, no sizable precommitted molecular repertoire will be found to explain cell–cell interaction in the developing nervous system.

6. Correlations will be found that suggest phased reentrant signaling on degenerate neuronal groups with periods of 50–200 msec. The most likely correlations will be found between cortical, thalamo-cortical, and limbic-reticular signals.

The theory will be falsified if any of the following conditions are found to hold:

1. Single cells are capable alone of "abstracting" sensory input in temporal or frontal cortex.

2. Removal of any single cell or distant combination of single cells relevant to a higher function results in loss of that function.

3. CNS cell groups are merely isomorphically and isofunc-tionally redundant but not degenerate.

4. Degenerate cell groups are found, but in such small numbers or restricted locales that their presence cannot account for a repertoire having both range and specificity. For example, if a total of only 10^3 groups were present for higher-order (R of R) processing of sensory modalities, it would be highly unlikely that they could carry out a wide range of different recognition functions.

5. The function of intrinsic connectivity within cell groups in the cortex and limbic areas (and possibly thalamic areas) is found to be completely fixed and determinate.

6. Evidence is obtained to rule out the presence of phasic re-entrant signaling.

Summary

A review of the properties of the central nervous system in higher mammals and particularly in man suggests that an adequate brain theory must account for the distributed nature of learning, the associative nature of recall, the adaptive reaction to novelty, and the capacity to make highly abstract representations in a world model. A selective theory of brain function in which the unit of selection is a neuronal group appears to account satisfactorily for these properties.

In the theory, it is assumed that structured neuronal groups containing up to 10,000 neurons are formed during embryogenesis and development. The intrinsic connections within a group and extrinsic connections among groups are specified by gene programming and synaptic selection. Upon completion of this process, primary repertoires are formed from neuronal groups of different structures and connectivity, more than one of which can respond to or recognize a particular signal pattern. This many-one response implies that each repertoire is degenerate. The polling of such degenerate primary repertoires by signals leads to associative recognition. Moreover, repetition of signals interacting with selected neuronal groups results in the emergence of secondary repertoires of groups with a higher likelihood of response. Such a process is selective in the sense that the signals play no role in the formation of anatomical connections within groups of the primary repertoire but only select appropriate groups from the preformed repertoire.

This selective theory of higher brain function requires no special thermodynamic assumptions and is free of mentalistic notions. Because the proposed system is selective and degenerate, however, it is not mechanistically determined in the sense that a clockwork machine is determined. On the basis of group-degenerate selection, an effort is made to account for the properties of consciousness by a phenomenological theory consistent with neuroanatomy and neurophysiology. The properties of consciousness to be accounted for include (1) the ability to appreciate or distinguish different events; (2) the capacity to react critically to inner or outer states and to update information; (3) the ability to accumulate memories and to recall them associatively in temporal sequences; and (4) the capacity to distinguish self from nonself (self-awareness). A satisfactory hypothesis accounting for these properties must avoid an infinite regression of hierarchical states and must provide for anticipatory planning and motor output without a programmer; that is, it must mitigate the need for programming.

The hypothesis advanced here is that the conscious state results from phasic reentrant signaling occurring in parallel processes that involve associations between stored patterns and current sensory or internal input. Each phasic process has two stages. The first stage consists of entry of processed input and holding of the resultant and associated signals for reentry into the second stage. In this stage, a subsequent processed input signal is linked with the reentrant signals and associated with the responses of groups in both primary and secondary repertoires. This cycle is completed in periods of milliseconds. Awareness is assumed to arise as a result of the access by groups of higher-order neurons to rich multimodal associative patterns stored in long-term memory as a result of past experience.

In this theory, the time base of reentry and that of recall are assumed to involve the same clock cycles. In concert with the sequential tagging of stored events, this allows for recall in a proper time scale and order. Because of the selective, group-degenerate, and phasic nature of reentrant cycles and the capacity of higher-order neurons to abstract sequences of events, a continuous shifting pattern of associations can be made. After sufficient development and experience, such a system can become capable of distinguishing abstract complexes such as the "self" from environmental input. Although this system is not dependent upon a fixed program or programmer, its properties are consistent with the ability of the brain to carry out complex routines.

According to this view, consciousness is considered to be a form of associative recollection with updating, based on present reentrant input, that continually confirms or alters a "world model" or "self theory" by means of parallel motor or sensory outputs. The entire process depends upon the properties of group selection and reentrant signaling in a nervous system that is already specified by embryological, developmental, and evolutionary events.

Acknowledgments

I am grateful to Francis O. Schmitt for his generous encouragement and valuable criticism, without which this paper would not have been written. My thanks are also due to Vernon Mountcastle whose expertise and judgment were invaluable during its preparation. The main argument of this paper remains my responsibility, however, and I assume the burden of any faults that may have escaped their notice.

References

Barondes, S., ed., 1976. *Neuronal Recognition*. New York: Plenum Press.

Bennett, T.L., 1975. The electrical activity of the hippocampus and the process of attention. In *The Hippocampus: Neurophysiology and Behavior*, Vol. 2, R.L. Isaacson and K.H. Pribram, eds. New York: Plenum Press.

Blakemore, C., and R.C. Van Sluyters, 1974. Reversal of the physiological effects of monocular deprivation in kittens: Further evidence for a sensitive period. *J. Physiol.* 237:195–216.

Bodian, D., 1970. A model of synaptic and behavioral ontogeny. In *The Neurosciences: Second Study Program*, F.O. Schmitt, ed. New York: The Rockefeller University Press, pp. 129–140.

Bodian, D., 1962. The generalized vertebrate neuron. *Science* 137:323–326.

Brackenbury, R., J.-P. Thiery, U. Rutishauser, and G.M. Edelman, 1977. Adhesion among neural cells of the chick embryo. I. An immunological assay for molecules involved in cell-cell binding. *J. Biol. Chem.*, 252:6835–6840.

Brodal, S., 1975. The "wiring patterns" of the brain: Neuroanatomical experiences and their implications for general views of the organization of the brain. In *The Neurosciences: Paths of Discovery*, F.G. Worden, J.P. Swazey, and G. Adelman, eds. Cambridge, Mass.: MIT Press, pp. 123–140.

Bullock, T.H., 1959. Neuron doctrine and electrophysiology. *Science* 129:997–1002.

Bullock, T.H., 1961. The problem of recognition in an analyzer made of neurons. In *Sensory Communication*, W.A. Rosenblith, ed. Cambridge, Mass.: MIT Press, pp. 717–724.

Bullock, T.H., and G.A. Horridge, 1965. *Structure and Function in the Nervous Systems of Invertebrates*, Vols. I and II. San Francisco: W.H. Freeman.

Campbell, K., 1970. *Body and Mind*. New York: Anchor Books, Doubleday and Co.

Changeux, J.-P., and A. Danchin, 1976. Selective stabilization of developing synapses as a mechanism for the specification of neuronal networks. *Nature* 264:705–712.

Chow, K.L., and A.L. Leiman, 1970. The structural and functional organization of the neocortex. *Neurosci. Res. Program Bull.* 8, No. 2.

Cooper, L.N., 1973. A possible organization of animal memory and learning. *Nobel Symposium* 24:252–264.

Cowan, W.M., 1973. Neuronal death as a regulative mechanism in the control of cell number in the nervous system. In *Development and Aging in the Nervous System*, M. Rockstein and M.L. Sussman, eds. New York: Academic Press, pp. 19–41.

Eccles, J.C., ed., 1966a. *Brain and Conscious Experience*. New York: Springer-Verlag.

Eccles, J.C., 1966b. Cerebral synaptic mechanisms. In *Brain and Conscious Experience*, J.C. Eccles, ed. New York: Springer-Verlag, pp. 24–50.

Eccles, J.C., 1974. Cerebral activity and consciousness. In *Studies in the Philosophy of Biology – Reduction and Related Problems*, F.J. Ayala and T. Dobzhansky, eds. London: Macmillan, pp. 87–105.

Edelman, G.M., 1974a. The problem of molecular recognition by a selective system. In *Studies in the Philosophy of Biology – Reduction and Related Problems*, F.J. Ayala and T. Dobzhansky, eds. London: Macmillan, pp. 45–56.

Edelman, G.M., 1974b. Origins and mechanisms of specificity in clonal selection. In *Cellular Selection and Regulation in the Immune Response*, G.M. Edelman, ed. New York: Raven Press.

Edelman, G.M., 1975. Molecular recognition in the immune and nervous systems. In *The Neurosciences: Paths of Discovery*, F.G. Worden, J.P. Swazey, and G. Adelman, eds. Cambridge, Mass.: MIT Press, pp. 65–74.

Evarts, V., E. Bizzi, R.E. Burke, M. DeLong, and W.T. Thach, Jr., 1971. Central control of movement. *Neurosci. Res. Program Bull.* 9, No. 1.

Feigl, H., 1967. *The "Mental" and the "Physical": The Essay and a Postscript.* Minneapolis: University of Minnesota Press.

Griffin, D., 1977. *The Question of Animal Awareness.* New York: Rockefeller University Press.

Grüsser, O.-J., and U. Grüsser-Cornehls, 1976. Neurophysiology of anuran visual system. In *Frog Neurobiology, A Handbook*, R. Llinás and W. Precht, eds. Berlin: Springer-Verlag, pp. 297–385.

Hamburger, V., 1970. Embryonic motility in vertebrates. In *The Neurosciences: Second Study Program*, F.O. Schmitt, ed. New York: The Rockefeller University Press, pp. 141–151.

Herrnstein, R.J., and E.G. Bornig, 1965. *A Source Book in the History of Psychology.* Cambridge, Mass.: Harvard University Press.

Hubel, D.H., and T.N. Wiesel, 1974. Sequence regularity and geometry of orientation columns in the monkey striate cortex. *J. Comp. Neurol.* 158:267–294.

Isaacson, R.L., and K.H. Pribram, eds., 1975a. *The Hippocampus: Structure and Development*, Vol. 1. New York: Plenum Press.

Isaacson, R.L., and K.H. Pribram, eds., 1975b. *The Hippocampus: Structure and Development*, Vol. 2, New York: Plenum Press.

Jasper, H.H., 1966. Pathophysiological studies of brain mechanisms in different states of consciousness. In *Brain and Conscious Experience*, J.C. Eccles, ed. New York: Springer-Verlag, pp. 256–282.

Jerne, N.K., 1967. Antibodies and learning: Selection versus instruction. In *The Neurosciences: A Study Program*, G.C. Quarton, T. Melnechuk, and F.O. Schmitt, eds. New York: The Rockefeller University Press, pp. 200–208.

Kandel, E., 1976. *Cellular Basis of Behavior.* San Francisco: W.H. Freeman.

Kuffler, S.W., and J.G. Nicholls, 1977. *From Neuron to Brain*. Sunderland, Mass.: Sinauer Associates, Inc.

Landmesser, L., and G. Pilar, 1970. Selective reinnervation of two cell populations in the adult pigeon ciliary ganglion. *J. Physiol*. 211:203–216.

Landmesser, L., and G. Pilar, 1972. The onset and development of transmission in the chick ciliary ganglion. *J. Physiol*. 222:691–713.

Lashley, K., 1950. In search of the engram. In *Physiological Mechanisms in Animal Behavior* (Society of Experimental Biology Symposium, No. 4). New York: Academic Press, pp. 454–482.

Lenneberg, E.H., 1970. Brain correlates of language. In *The Neurosciences: Second Study Program*, F.O. Schmitt, ed. New York: The Rockefeller University Press, pp. 361–371.

Libet, B., 1966. Brain stimulation and the threshold of conscious experience. In *Brain and Conscious Experience*, J.C. Eccles, ed. New York: Springer-Verlag, pp. 165–176.

Longuet-Higgins, H.C., D.J. Willshaw, and O.P. Berneman, 1970. Theories of associative recall. *Quart. Rev. Biophys*. 3, No. 2.

Luria, A.R., 1973. *The Working Brain: An Introduction to Neuropsychology*. New York: Basic Books.

MacKay, D.M., 1966. Cerebral organization and the conscious control of action. In *Brain and Conscious Experience*, J.C. Eccles, ed. New York: Springer-Verlag, pp. 422–445.

MacKay, D.M., 1970. Perception and brain function. In *The Neurosciences: Second Study Program*, F.O. Schmitt, ed. New York: The Rockefeller University Press, pp. 303–316.

Miller, G.A., and P.N. Johnson-Laird, 1976. *Language and Perception*. Cambridge, Mass.: Harvard University Press.

Moscona, A., 1974. Surface specification of embryonic cells: Lectin receptors, cell recognition and specific cell ligands. In *The Cell Surface in Development*, A. Moscona, ed. New York: John Wiley & Sons.

Mountcastle, V.B., 1957. Modality and topographic properties of single neurons of cat's somatic sensory cortex. *J. Neurophysiol*. 20:408–434.

Mountcastle, V.B., 1967. The problems of sensing and the neural coding of sensory events. In *The Neurosciences: A Study Program*, G.C. Quarton, T. Melnechuk, and F.O. Schmitt, eds. New York: The Rockefeller University Press, pp. 393–408.

Mountcastle, V.B., 1974. Sleep, wakefulness, and the conscious state: Intrinsic regulatory mechanisms of the brain. In *Medical Physiology*, Vol. 1, V.B. Mountcastle, ed. St. Louis: C.V. Mosby Co., pp. 254–281.

Mountcastle, V.B., 1976. The world around us: Neural command functions for selective attention. *Neurosci. Res. Program Bull*. 14, Supplement.

Nauta, W.J.H., and H.J. Karten, 1970. A general profile of the vertebrate brain with sidelights on the ancestry of the cerebral cortex. In *The Neurosciences: Second Study Program*, F.O. Schmitt, ed. New York: The Rockefeller University Press, pp. 7–26.

Penfield, W., 1975. The mind and the brain. In *The Neurosciences: Paths of Discovery*, F.G. Worden, J.P. Swazey, and G. Adelman, eds. Cambridge, Mass.: MIT Press, pp. 437–454.

Peters, A., S.L. Palay, and H. dé F. Webster, 1976. *The Fine Structure of the Nervous System*. Philadelphia: Saunders.

Piaget, J., 1950. *Psychology of Intelligence*, New York: Harcourt, Brace and World.

Piaget, J., 1954. *The Construction of Reality in the Child*. New York: Basic Books.

Popper, K.R., 1974. Scientific reduction and the essential incompleteness of all science. In *Studies in Philosophy of Biology—Reduction and Related Problems*, F.J. Ayala and T. Dobzhansky, eds. London: Macmillan, pp. 259–283.

Prestige, H.C., 1970. Differentiation, degeneration, and the role of the periphery. In *The Neurosciences: Second Study Program*, F.O. Schmitt, ed. New York: The Rockefeller University Press, pp. 73–82.

Pribram, K.H., and R.L. Isaacson, 1975. Summary. In *The Hippocampus: Neurophysiology and Behavior*, Vol. 2, R.L. Isaacson and K.H. Pribram, eds. New York: Plenum Press, pp. 429–441.

Quarton, G.C., T. Melnechuk, and F.O. Schmitt, eds., 1967. *The Neurosciences: A Study Program*. New York: The Rockefeller University Press.

Rakic, P., 1975. Local circuit neurons. *Neurosci. Res. Program Bull.* 13, No. 2.

Russell, W.R., and M.L.E. Espir, 1961. *Traumatic Aphasia*. London: Oxford University Press.

Ryle, G., 1949. *The Concept of Mind*. New York: Barnes and Noble.

Schmitt, F.O., ed., 1970. *The Neurosciences: Second Study Program*. New York: The Rockefeller University Press.

Schmitt, F.O., and F.G. Worden, eds., 1974. *The Neurosciences: Third Study Program*. Cambridge, Mass.: MIT Press.

Schmitt, F.O., P. Dev, and B.H. Smith, 1976. Electrotonic processing of information by brain cells. *Science* 193:114–120.

Seckel, H.P.G., 1950. *Bird Headed Dwarfs*. Springfield, Ill.: Charles C Thomas.

Shepherd, G.M., 1972. The neuron doctrine: A revision of functional concepts. *Yale J. Biol. Med.* 45:584–599.

Sherrington, C.S., 1941. *Man on His Nature*. Cambridge, England: Cambridge University Press.

Skinner, B.F., 1966. The phylogeny and ontogeny of behavior. *Science* 153:1205–1213.

Sperry, R.W., 1969. A modified concept of consciousness. *Psychol. Rev.* 76:532–536.

Sperry, R.W., 1970a. Perception in the absence of the neocortical commissures. In *Perception and Its Disorders*, D.A. Hamburg, K.H. Pribram, and A.J. Stunkard, eds. Baltimore: William & Wilkins, pp. 123–138.

Sperry, R.W., 1970b. An objective approach to subjective experience. *Psychol. Rev.* 77:585–590.

Thiery, J.-P., R. Brackenbury, U. Rutishauser, and G.M. Edelman, 1977. Adhesion among neural cells of the chick embryo. II. Purification and characterization of a cell adhesion molecule from neural retina. *J. Biol. Chem.* 252:6841–6845.

Vanderwolf, C.H., R. Krassies, L.A. Gillespie, and B.H. Blond, 1975. Hippocampal rhythmic slow activity and neocortical low voltage fast activity: Relations to behavior. In *The Hippocampus: Neurophysiology and Behavior*, Vol. 2, R.L. Isaacson and K.H. Pribram, eds. New York: Plenum Press, pp. 101–128.

Vinogradova, O.S., 1975. Functional organization of the limbic system in the process of the registration of information: Facts and hypotheses. In *The Hippocampus: Neurophysiology and Behavior*, Vol. 2, R.L. Isaacson and K.H. Pribram, eds. New York: Plenum Press, pp. 3–69.

von Neumann, J., 1956. Probabilistic logics and the synthesis of reliable organisms from unreliable components. In *Automata Studies*, C. Shannon and J. McCarthy, eds. Princeton: Princeton University Press, pp. 43–98.

Weiss, P., 1970. Neural development in biological perspective. In *The Neurosciences: Second Study Program*, F.O. Schmitt, ed. New York: The Rockefeller University Press, pp. 53–61.

Wilson, D.M., 1970. Neural operations in arthropod ganglia. In *The Neurosciences: Second Study Program*, F.O. Schmitt, ed. New York: The Rockefeller University Press, pp. 397–409.

Wilson, H.R., and J.D. Cowan, 1973. A mathematical theory of the functional dynamics of cortical and thalamic nervous tissue. *Kyternetik* 13:55–80.

Winograd, S., and J.D. Cowan, 1963. *Reliable Computations in the Presence of Noise.* Cambridge, Mass.: MIT Press.

Yoon, M.G., 1975. Topographic polarity of the optic tectum studied by reimplantation of the tectal tissue in adult goldfish. In *Cold Spring Harbor Symposia on Quantitative Biology*, Vol. XL, New York: Cold Spring Harbor Laboratory, pp. 503–519.

Young, J.Z., 1975. Sources of discovery in neuroscience. In *The Neurosciences: Paths of Discovery*, F.G. Worden, J.P. Swazey, and G. Adelman, eds. Cambridge, Mass.: MIT Press, pp. 15–46.

Printed in the United States
by Baker & Taylor Publisher Services

Printed in the United States
by Baker & Taylor Publisher Services